THE WATER OF LIFE

THE WATER OF LIFE

A Treatise on Urine-Therapy

by

JOHN W. ARMSTRONG

THE C.W. DANIEL CO. LTD.
1 Church Path, Saffron Walden,
Essex, England

Second Edition
Second Impression 1971
Third Impression 1974
Fourth Impression 1976
Fifth Impression 1978
Sixth Impression 1981
Seventh Impression 1984
Eighth Impression 1987
Ninth Impression 1990
Tenth Impression 1993
Eleventh Impression 1995
Twelfth Impression 1998

© THE C.W. DANIEL CO. LTD. 1971

ISBN 0 85032 052 6

Produced in Great Britain by
PRINT MATTERS 01279 302095

CONTENTS

FOREWORD

By those many people who have derived and are still deriving benefit from Urine-Therapy I have repeatedly been asked to write a book, but hitherto I have demurred. First, because the necessary leisure has been lacking, and secondly, because I am averse to any form of self-advertisement. However, realising that a thing which is put off too long may never be accomplished at all, I have finally decided to yield to persuasions, and this treatise is largely compiled from notes, case-sheets and letters. Other reasons for giving out my experiences to the world will become apparent to the reader in due course. I am fully aware that the publication of a book is attended with certain indirect drawbacks; one is that the writer may be inundated with letters, and another is that, if he is a practitioner, he may be inundated with patients, who may apply to him c/o his publishers. As I am not touting for patients, that was a further reason why I wished to delay writing this book. But now that it is going forth to the public, the following must be emphasised :

(1) A law having been passed making it now illegal for any but a qualified medical practitioner to declare he can cure certain specific diseases—cancer being one— it should be noted that all case-histories relative to such diseases mentioned in this book are those of patients treated prior to the passing of the law in question. I am not in a position to state whether the law can be stretched so far as to make it illegal for a layman even to say he *has* cured such disorders in the past; but if so, then, in accordance with the medical dictum, one is forced to assume that where any such diseases have yielded to

7

other than orthodox treatment, they have perforce been wrongly diagnosed !

(2) As the therapy to be outlined in this book is an entirely drugless system of healing and is a specific for health and not for any given disease, diagnosis plays no practical part in the treatment. Thus, although the chapters are headed with the names of various disorders. it is merely for the sake of literary expedience and to show that they have proved amenable to the general treatment.

JOHN W. ARMSTRONG.

1944.

" Many people believe that fifty thousand doctors, vast hospitals, armies of nurses, dentists, chemists, clinics, and about three hundred thousand mentally deranged, are signs of progressive medicine and civilisation, but actually they demonstrate complete failure of our medical system, and wrong guidance of the public in nutrition and other ways of living. Thousands of operations carried out weekly with brilliant technique, give additional proof that the prior treatments had not achieved successful cure."

* * *

" Health and not disease is the true inheritance of life. Human creatures fail to realise facts which stare them in the face. We are made of what we eat, so if any organ becomes diseased, it generally means the food was wrong. . . . ."

MAJOR C. FRASER MACKENZIE, C.I.E.
(Health Through Homœopathy, June, July, 1944).

" Disease . . . . becomes a vested interest, and consciously or unconsciously, the doctors foster it as such. It is quite a common observation that doctors produce disease. Moreover, the whole system and philosophy of our dealing with disease is mistaken."

DR. W. H. WHITE, M.R.C.S., L.R.C.P.

Hippocrates, the great priest of medicine, advised the physicians to accept the help of the laity in the treatment of disease, but his advice has seldom been followed.

Like the kingdom of heaven, the kingdom of health has to be taken by storm.

J.W.A.

CHAPTER I.

INTRODUCTION

Owing to the increasing part played by vested interests in many branches of human endeavour, not least in the very lucrative providing of remedies for disease, intelligent members of the public are growing more and more distrustful of orthodox medical methods. Many people must have asked themselves the following questions :

How comes it that for over fifty years the orthodox cancer researchers have been occupying themselves with the cause and cure of malignancy, yet still can suggest nothing better than the knife, radium or X-rays?

How comes it that *after* letters from many doctors had appeared in the *British Medical Journal* testifying to the highly unsatisfactory results of radium treatment, it is none the less still boosted in this country and elsewhere?

How comes it that when effective treatments for cancer have been discovered either by a qualified doctor or by practitioners of unorthodox schools, they have not been recognised by the Cancer Research Ring, which still asks the public to donate large sums towards the discovery of a cure?

To these questions (with which I shall deal in my Afterword) no satisfactory answers are forthcoming, and we are forced to the conclusion that, although there are many selfless and noble-minded doctors to be found in most countries, in modern Medicine itself many things prevail which are much to be deplored. (1) The torture of animals for experimentation and for the preparation

10

of sera and vaccines ; (2) the fostering of fear in the public mind by means of advertising ; (3) commercialism and vested interests which ought to play no part in healing the sick ; and (4) a narrow spirited element of trade unionism which suggests that the patients exist for the doctors instead of vice versa : all these things many doctors themselves have at one time or another commented upon and regretted in forcible terms.

And yet, as after a war, Nature or " the Higher Powers " seem to step in to adjust the balance of things by insuring that a greater proportion of male children should be born, so when Medicine becomes over-tinctured with material considerations do they seem to inspire some method of healing as a corrective to these tendencies, and as a help to those who are large-minded enough to take advantage of it. Such a method may be precluded by other methods which prepare the way for its acceptance ; for one must admit that naturopathy has been instrumental in curing many diseases where the orthodox system has signally failed. Nevertheless, as we shall see anon, naturopathy as it is usually practised does not go far enough, for although it can cleanse the body of its toxins, it cannot replace wasted tissues incidental to such grievous ills as consumption or other diseases of equal gravity. This can only be accomplished by an elaboration of an ancient therapy, the details of which I propose to put forward in this book, and which I have practised on myself and some thousands of others with signal success, although many of them were said to be suffering from incurable diseases. It is true that at one time I had resolved not to write my book until I had had the chance of curing even leprosy ; but as I am unlikely to come across a case of this dread disease unless enabled to visit those countries where it is prevalent, I have decided to give the details of my experiences to the public without further delay. My contention is—and I do not stand

11

alone in putting it forward—that within Man himself is to be found the substance to cure his diseases, whether they be so-called wasting diseases or otherwise ; and I propose to substantiate this contention by case-sheets, on the principle that one ounce of facts is worth many pounds of theories

If in the course of stating the facts, references to medical failures should be essential, this is unavoidable in the interests of the public and of truth itself ; and such references are made in no spirit of hostility towards doctors.   As already implied there are many unselfish and honest physicians to whom I wish to do no injustice : it is erroneous and harmful beliefs and practices* which I am constrained to criticise, *not* personalities. The readers will see for themselves that such criticism cannot arise from any ulterior motives.   I have no secret remedy or patent medicine to sell.   Indeed, although a layman, I am only following the policy required from all reputable members of the .Medical Profession themselves, viz., to make no secret of any discovery which may prove useful in curing mankind : the more so as in many cases the treatment can be carried out at home without any financial outlay whatever.

* This aspect of the matter has been fully dealt with by Mr.
  Ellis Barker (whose books are published by John Murray)
  and by Mr. Cyril Scott in his *Doctors, Disease and Health*
  and *Victory Over Cancer; The Cauldron of Disease* by Are
  Waerland, also repays study.

CHAPTER II.

THE WATER OF LIFE

Before relating my own experiences with urine-therapy, it is advisable to quote some opinions derived from both ancient and modern sources as to the value of urine as a curative agent.

Towards the beginning of last century, a book entitled *One Thousand Notable Things* was published simultaneously in England, Scotland and Ireland. In this book appeared the following quaint citation :

" An universal and excellent remedy for all distempers inward and outward—Drink you own water in the morning nine days together and it cures the scurvy, makes the body lightsome and cheerful.

" It is good against the dropsy and jaundice, drunk as before (stated).

" Wash your ears with it warm and it is good against deafness, noises and most other ailments in the ears.

" Wash your eyes with your own water and it cures sore eyes and clears and strengthens the sight.

" Wash and rub your hands with it and it takes away numbness, chaps and sores and makes the joints limber.

" Wash any green wound with it and it is an extraordinary good thing.

" Wash any part that itches and it takes it (the itch) away.

" Wash the fundament and it is good against piles and other sores."

Here is another quaintly expressed extract from an old book called *Salmon's English Physician*, published in 1695, which I will quote in part :

" Urine is taken from human kind and most four-footed animals ; but the former is that which is chiefly used in Physick and Chemistry. It is the serum or watery part of the blood, which being diverted by the emulgent arteries to the reins is there separated, and by the ferment of the parts, converted into urine .... Man's or woman's urine is hot, dry (?), dissolving, cleansing, discussing, resists putrefaction ; used inwardly against obstructions of the liver, spleen, gall, as also against the Dropsie, Jaundice, Stoppage of the terms in women, the Plague and all manner of malign fevers. . . . .

" Outwardly (applied) it cleanses the skin and softens it by washing it therewith, especially being warm, or new made. Cleanses, heals and dries up wounds, though made with poisoned weapons. Cures dandruff, scurf, and bathed upon the pulses, cools the heat of fevers. Is excellent against trembling, numbness and the palsy, and bathed upon the region of the spleen, urine eases the pains thereof.

"The virtues of the volatile salts of urine—It powerfully absorbs acids and destroys the very root of most diseases in human bodies. It opens all obstructions of . . . . Reins, Mysentery and Womb, purifies the whole mass of Blood and Humors cures . . . Caclexia . . . Rheumatism and Hypochrondriac diseases, and is given with admirable success in Epilepsies, Vertigoes, Apoplexies, Convulsions, Lythargies, Migraine, Palsies, Lameness, Numbness, loss of the use of limbs, atrophies, vapors, fits of the mother, and most cold and moist diseases of the head, brain, nerves, joints and womb. (Leucorrhoea should be added to this list.)

" It opens obstructions of the reins and urinary passages, dissolves tartarous coagulations in those parts, breaks and expels stone and gravel.

" It is a specific remedy against Dysuria, Ischuria and all obstructions of Urine whatsoever."

So much for this panegyric on what some of us have come to term *the eau de vie.* But one also reads that in the 18th century it was much extolled as a valuable mouth-wash by a Parisian dentist.

I will now quote some modern opinions as to the value of urine.

Writing in *Candide,* Prof. Jean Rostande repeatedly stresses the biological significance of those substances known as hormones. The gist of his article of some 1.250 words may be condensed as follows :

" A recent discovery regarding the activity of hormones has completely revolutionised their study—viz.. that certain of them filter through the kidney to pass out in the urine. Multiple hypophysical hormones, the hormones of the adrenal and hormones of the sexual glands, have been found in normal urine . . . The discovery of hormone-urinoltogy has had far-reaching consequences. Urine provides a practically unlimited quantity of basic matter. . . . From the therapeutic point of view it is possible to envisage the use of these human hormones as apparently capable of exercising great power over the human organism . . . ."

Thus urine extolled by many of the ancients, but misunderstood by the semi-moderns, now appears in the light of a wonderful reservoir—a philtre of pre-eminent value. It contains in a pure and often undreamt of quantity, products of the most vital nature, bearing out what Mr. Ellis Barker maintained when he wrote that " our body distils the most wonderful medicines and provides the most perfect serums and anti-bodies."

I will now quote some remarks taken from a pamphlet by Dr. T. Wilson Deachman, Ph.C., M.D., who writes :

15

" As the urine content varies according to the pathological state of the patient, its use is indicated in all forms of disease except those caused by traumatism (broken limbs) or those that are of a mechanical nature. It saves the physician from the mistake that is made in selecting the indicated remedy from three thousand drugs or more. . . . What cannot be cured by the forces of the body cannot be cured by the forces outside the body."

It is not irrelevant here to mention that the late Maurice Wilson, who made a magnificent, if abortive, attempt to climb Mount Everest, ascribed his immunity from ordinary ills and his astonishing stamina to his many fasts on urine only, plus external friction with urine. 1. ; Llamas of Thibet and the yogis with whom he associated prior to his attempt, claim to live to a great age by means of the use of urine. By the same means they can also traverse deserts inaccessible to ordinary mortals.

Last century, between the eighteen-sixties to seventies, the drinking of one's own urine was a well-known cure for jaundice, and some doctors had the courage to prescribe it. I learned from one of my patients that, when he was a boy, his grandfather had cured him of an attack of jaundice by urging him, on the advice of a doctor, to drink all the urine he passed during the four days of his illness.

Among gipsies, the health-giving properties of urine have been known for centuries. Cow's urine has been taken in large quantities for the cure of Bright's disease, dropsy and other afflictions. I once met a Dorset farmer who had over a period of sixty years drunk four pints of cow's urine a day. He was 80 at the time, straight as a yard-stick, and he told me that he was never ill. He had, on the advice of a gipsy, begun the treatment at the age of 20 for throat and chest trouble. Nevertheless,

16

cow's urine as a curative agent is inferior to the patient's own urine, and I have known it to fail in a case of Bright's disease brought on by alcoholism.

The wiser of the ancient Greeks used nothing but urine for the treatment of wounds. The Eskimos even to this day adopt the same measures.

The question may be asked if urine-therapy has been used by anyone in comparatively recent times? And the answer is in the affirmative. Apart from others, the late W. H. Baxter, J.P., of Leeds and Harrogate, not only took his own urine, but wrote numerous pamphlets on the subject which might have been regarded more seriously had they not been interlarded with somewhat irrelevant moralisings. " Mr. Baxter, who lived to a ripe old age, declaring that he had cured himself of a cancerous growth by applying his own urine in the form of compresses, and by drinking his own urine neat. He further declared that he had cured himself of other complaints by these simple means. Mr. Baxter contended that urine is the finest antiseptic that exists, and, having made this discovery, he formed the daily habit of drinking three tumblers full as a prophylactic against disease. He maintained that if autogenous urine is taken in this way, the more innocuous it becomes. He applied it to his eyes as a strengthening lotion, and used it, after shaving, for his complexion. He also advocated its external use for wounds, swellings, boils, etc. As an aperient he declared it to be unsurpassed." (See *Doctors, Disease and Health,* by Cyril Scott.)

I can vouch for the truth of this statement, as Mr. Baxter was for a short time one of my patients. But what is not mentioned in the above is that during the treatment he *fasted* on urine and water only. This fasting, as the reader will see later, is an essential part of the treatment—at any rate in serious disease conditions.

17

In some rural districts the use of cow's urine has been advocated by doctors for boils. A case may be quoted of a man who had a number of painful boils under his arm. They were quickly cured by compresses of cow's urine.

En passant, I may mention that not so long ago one of the most exclusive and expensive toilet soaps was made from the dehydrated salts and fats of the urine of grass-fed cows, and another from the urine of Russian peasants. (My informant was a chemist who knew what he was talking about.) Furthermore some expensive face-creams contain hormones derived from human urine. " What the eye seeth not. . . ." !

CHAPTER III.

SOME OBJECTIONS ANSWERED

Before proceeding, it is advisable to deal with some objections which have been, and may still be, raised. It has been argued that if man were intended to drink his own urine he would have been born with the instinct to do so. But one may as well argue that because man has not been born with the instinct to do deep breathing exercises or adopt other measures which have proved conducive to health, they are therefore invalid or reprehensible. Take, for instance, the yogis of India. By dint of practising breathing exercises, strange postures, etc., they not only arrive at a perfect state of health, but contrive to extend life far beyond the usual three score years and ten. At 150 years of age a proficient Hatha Yogi has not even a grey hair. (See *Rajah Yoga*, by Swami Vivikananda.) It is true that the science of Yoga can only be safely learnt at the hands of a competent teacher ; but that is another argument against the instinct theory. (See *Heaven Lies Within Us* by Theos Bernard.) One notices, by the way, that man does not trouble about his instincts when it is a question of imbibing strong liquors, or smoking hundreds of cigarettes : in short, when it is a matter of doing things which are bad for him even though the first time he experienced their " delights " his instinct rebelled.

And now to answer another objection. How can it be right to take back into the body something which the body is apparently discarding? And yet if we turn to Nature, what do we find? We find that where instead of " scientific " manures, the dead leaves are put back into the soil, the resultant flowers are the most fragrant, the fruits the sweeter, and the trees the healthier. On the other hand, where the soil is for some reason deprived of those chemical substances produced by the dead leaves, etc., then the trees which grow in that soil are disfigured by excrescences, which I think, quite aptly have been called tree-cancers. What we are accustomed to regard as useless dead leaves are the very opposite of useless, and should be dug back into the soil instead of being swept away by the gardener. Let those who challenge this statement taste the *Iceni* Produce, grown from soil treated on the principle that all that comes from the soil should be put back into the soil, and they will soon be convinced that the principle is a correct one. The idea that Nature is wasteful is erroneous. She only appears wasteful to us because we do not understand her. The rotting dead leaves provide the most valuable mineral salts for the soil—one of the most essential being potash. Even the ashes of burnt dead leaves and burnt wood (charcoal) are of great value. Therefore why should a principle which applies throughout Nature not apply (with certain reservations) to the human body? This question is the more readily answered if we consider the constituents of urine.

Yet before doing so, something should be said about the unreliability of urine analysis as a means of diagnosis. Though urine-analysis is still a practice among orthodox doctors, it has been found that the elements in and general condition of urine depend far more on the character of the food and drink taken by the patient than on any fancied or real disease condition. Even the presence of sugar can no longer be regarded as an infallible sign of diabetes. This I have proved to my own satisfaction by taking for a day nothing but drinks made of chemical sweet powders, and nothing in the way of food except a quantity of heavily sweetened ices. On such a diet, after twelve to fourteen hours the urine of an otherwise healthy person became charged with sugar and suggested to the doctor that he had diabetes! Similar mistakes have been made with regard to albumen found in the urine as the result of an ill-balanced diet. Some years ago a friend of the writer's connected with a Life Insurance Company had a number of "prospects" turned down owing to heavy deposits of albumen in their urine. Finally he brought three of these men along for investigation. By dint of altering their diet, all the supposed-to-be indications of Bright's disease, nephritis or albuminuria from which they were alleged to be suffering very soon vanished, and at a subsequent examination by the Insurance doctor they were told they must have had "local inflammations" when previously examined! Further comment seems superfluous.

Urea N. (nitrogen)	682
Urea	1459
Creatinine N.	36
Creatinine	97.2
Uric acid N.	12.3
Uric acid	36.9
Amino N.	9.7
Ammonia N.	57
Sodium	212
Potassium	137
Calcium	19.5
Magnesium	11.3
Chloride	314
Total sulphate	91
Inorganic sulphate	83

Inorganic phosphate	127
pH	6.4
Total acidity as C.C.	
N/10 acid	27.8 *

This is significant as showing the amount of valuable mineral salts contained in healthy urine ; to appreciate which, one needs to have studied The Biochemic System of Medicine. Even so, as already implied, there are wide variations in urinary composition according to the foods and drinks consumed. For instance, taking fifty normal subjects, we find that whereas with the average, Urea N. amounts to 682, the maximum amounts to 1829, whilst the minimum is 298. As to the volume of urine passed, it varies greatly according to diet and season of the year. Also, urine passed at night is about one quarter to one half of that passed during daytime.

In view of the above analysis, we may well ask ourselves the question : If the elements which urine reveals are not required by the body, then why do our food chemists and biochemists emphasise their value and declare them to be essential to the body upkeep?

The idea that urine contains poisonous elements which the body is endeavouring to eliminate is based upon theory only, and is not demonstrated by the facts. As survivors in open boats and rafts often drink their own urine when their water supply becomes deficient, surely if they were drinking a poisonous fluid they would die or become very ill? Far from this being the case, the practice of drinking urine is pronounced to be harmless. but (as the Medical Department of the Navy pointed out in a letter to an inquirer) " the benefit obtained is not as great as would appear at first sight because in dehydration the output of urine falls to a very low level. . : ." I shall comment on this later. Meanwhile, I may remark that what may be a " poison " when separated from its natural environment may not act as a poison when *remaining* in its natural environment. The Medical Profession may have been impressed when, at the beginning of the century, Charrin wrote a whole book on the " poisons " of urine, but as Prof. Jean Rostand (already quoted) has since written : " The time is not far off when it will be imperative to write of the blessings of urine." Indeed, as we shall see in the course of these pages, the most pregnant of all facts is the outstanding fact that urine, however thick, concentrated, scanty and seemingly " poisonous " it may appear at the onset of such diseases as genuine Bright's disease, influenza and others, very soon becomes filtered and greatly increased in volume when freely imbibed. This is a fact I have witnessed, together with other practitioners of urine-therapy, in hundreds of so-termed hopeless cases, and is the best and most definite answer to the objection with which I am dealing.

One other objection which has been mooted (namely by those who are wont to put their trust in the " princes " of medicine) is as follows : If urine was at one time known to be such a valuable remedy, why has it fallen into disrepute? And yet those who put this question must be unacquainted with the most elementary facts of orthodox medical history, which related of one long series of changes of policy, changes of drugs, of treatments, of fads and fashions and "exploded superstitions," of altercations, of envies and even of persecutions. Some of the strangest " remedies " have had a vogue for a few years, only to be regarded a few years later as the most disgusting and barbarous superstitions. For instance, the notorious Cardinal Richlieu was given horse-

23

dung in wine to drink on his death-bed, and not by quacks but by men we should nowadays call qualified doctors. (See *Devils, Drugs and Doctors,* by H. W. Haggard, MH.D.) Nor am I here giving away "state secrets" in alluding to the instability which characterises the orthodox Medical Profession. Speaking at the King's College H.M. School on October 1st, 1918, Surgeon-General Sir Watson Cheyne, M.P.. urged the students to remember :—

"Medicine is not an exact science. A good deal of what they were being taught was not true. When they came to deal with life, they knew so little about the living body that they could not be dogmatic. They could only lay down hypotheses which would hold for a day and then pass away : and just as the teachings of seventy years ago seemed to them very curious and not very sound, so it would be exactly the same forty years *hence." (The Times,* October 2nd, 1918.)

The truth of this utterance applies every bit as much to-day as it did in 1918—perhaps even more so. It is no exaggeration to say that, far from being an exact science, in spite of all " scientific " tests that patients are subjected to in these days, it still remains such an *in*exact science that ten different doctors have been known to give ten different diagnoses relative to so apparently simple an ailment as persistent headaches. In the American journal *Liberty* (January 22nd, 1938) there appeared a significant article by a man in the late twenties who relates his attempts to get rid of this annoying trouble by consulting no less than ten doctors in succession ; and at the end of his adventures he still retained his headaches. As the story is so significant and not unfraught with its ironic and humorous side, it may be condensed here.

The *first* doctor told him he had an obstruction in his

24

nose, and must see a nose specialist; the *second* told him
there was nothing the matter with his nose, but he must
see an oculist ; the *third* told him he had low blood
pressure, and must have injections ; the *fourth* told him
he had high blood pressure, and must diet himself to
lower it ; the *fifth* told him his liver was enlarged, and
he must have electrical treatment ; the *sixth* told him his
liver was not enlarged but it secreted insufficient bile ; the
seventh told him that his pituitary gland was not functioning properly, and he must have glandular injections :
the *eighth* told him he was suffering from intestinal
poisoning, and must cut down his eating and smoking ;
the *ninth* told him that his was a case of nervous debility,
and he must take some pills for the trouble, the *tenth*
told him there was nothing really the matter with him,
and that his headaches were just headaches ! . . . In
citing this article I am not implying that doctors are
ignoramuses.   On the contrary, they are so full of eru-
dition that " they cannot see the wood of truth for the
trees of learning " !   That is one very cogent reason why
sooner or later they reject the simple remedy or treatment
for the complex, no matter how efficacious that simple
remedy has proved to be.

A final objection which may be raised against urine
intake by the fastidious (although it constitutes no
argument against its therapeutical value) is that the taste
must be so " utterly revolting " that only heroes could
bring themselves to drink it.   This assumption, however,
is incorrect.   The taste of healthy urine is not nearly as
objectionable as, say, Epsom salts.   Fresh morning urine
is merely somewhat bitter and salty.   But as already
mentioned, the more frequently it is taken the more
innocuous does it become ; and as might be expected, its
taste varies from day to day and even from hour to hour
according to the foods which have been eaten.   Even the
urine which is passed in some serious diseases is not as
obnoxious to taste as its appearance may often suggest.

25

And now, having cited testimonials both ancient and modern as to the therapeutical value of urine, and having also dealt with the afore-mentioned objections, I will sum up the evidence contained through many years of practice and personal experience on the part of those who are in a position to know the real facts.

Urine, on being taken into the body, is filtered; it becomes purer and purer even in the course of one day's living upon it, plus tap-water, if required. First, it cleanses, then frees from obstruction and finally rebuilds the vital organs and passages after they have been wasted by the ravages of disease. In fact it rebuilds not only the lungs, pancreas, liver, brain, heart, etc., but also repairs the linings of brain and bowel and other linings, as has been demonstrated in the case of many "killing" diseases, such as consumption of the intestines and the worst form of colitis. In fine, it accomplishes what fasting merely on water or fruit juices (as some naturo-paths advocate) can never achieve.

The proof of this statement will be found in the case-histories adduced in the following pages.

CHAPTER IV.

My Self-Cure

Although I should prefer to avoid the first personal pronoun in this book, it is not possible to do so in the circumstances if I am to carry conviction. For, as already implied, one ounce of experience outweighs a ton of arguments !

My first patient was myself. It happened in this wise. During the last war at the age of thirty-four, I presented myself for medical examination under what was called The Derby Scheme, and was rejected by four examining doctors on the grounds that I was consumptive. Moreover I was urged to put myself under the care of a physician. Consequently I consulted a specialist. He however, treated my condition as not very serious, told me I was more a catarrhal subject than a consumptive one, and advised plenty of fresh air, sunshine and a nourishing diet. I followed his advice, and in one year put on 28lbs. in weight. Nevertheless, not being satisfied with my condition I consulted another specialist, who informed me that both my lungs were affected, and despite what the previous specialist had said, I *was* consumptive, and must keep up my strength on a diet rich in sugars and starches. Finally, diabetes set in, and I was placed on an entirely new and drastic regime, which consisted of fasting on six half-pints a day of cold water (sipped) during four days of every week, whilst on the fifth and two following days I was permitted a " snack " which only served to whet my appetite, not to mention the fact that I was enjoined to chew every morsel of it to such a degree that it only produced a very sore mouth, aching teeth, swollen gums and a swollen tongue. In

27

addition to these discomforts, I was inflicted with insomnia, frayed nerves, and great irritability of temper. The regime was continued for sixteen weeks without a break, and although it resulted in the disappearance of my cough and catarrhal conditions, and also of painful sciatica from which I had suffered, none the less the cure seemed more unpleasant to me than the disease. The final upshot was, that after two years of this treatment, I lost faith in doctors and began a series of ventures on my own, although much against their advice.

I will not prolong this story by giving all the details ; suffice it to say, there came a moment when, feeling very weak and ill, I recalled the text in Proverbs V. which runs, " Drink waters out of thine own cistern," a text which, in its turn, reminded me of the case of a young girl whose father gave her her own urine to drink when she was suffering from diphtheria, *with the result that he cured her in three days.* Other cases also came to mind (jaundice was one) which had been cured by the same means. Nor was this all ; I remembered the doctor's answer to my question when some few years previously I had asked him how he could tell from my urine that my lungs and pancreas were diseased and wasting? I even remembered saying to him in my then innocence : " If I am losing vital tissue and sugar through my urine, then why not drink the urine and replace these elements in that way? " To which he had replied that the organs could not assimilate " dead matter." This, however, as I have proved since, was nothing but a theoretical fallacy !

And here to digress for a moment. I grant that it is unwise dogmatically to assert that any given text of Scripture denotes this or that, for many people read into the Bible exactly what they themselves wish to find there. Nevertheless, I believed, and still believe, that the text I have quoted, and many others also, bear reference to that vital fluid which is within our own bodies ; and believing it, I acted in accordance with that belief, to find in the end that it proved to be my physical salvation. Fortified by my faith in what I thought to be the correct interpretation of the text, I fasted for forty-five days on nothing but urine and tap water—and this, despite the doctor's assertion that eleven days without food was the limit to which a human being could go : I also rubbed urine into my body—a very important factor in the cure, with which I shall deal in Chapter XVII—I finally broke my fast on raw beef, and though it gave me no discomfort beyond a ravenous hunger, I none the less ate cautiously for a time, and continued to drink my own urine, noticing that its changes in temperature, quantity, taste, etc., depended almost entirely on what I ate or drank, and on the amount of exercise I took.

At the end of this treatment I felt and was " an entirely new man." I weighed 140 lbs., was full of vim, looked about eleven years younger than I actually was, and had a skin like a young girl's. I was thirty-six at the time, and am now over sixty. Yet by dint of drinking every drop of water that I pass, living on a well-balanced diet,* and never eating more food *per diem* than I consider the body requires, I look and feel much younger than most men of my age, and keep free from those major and minor ailments to which the body is said to be heir.

Having now related the essential details of my self-cure and all that contributed to its continuance, I will merely add that in 1918, being convinced that knowledge must not be selfishly " hidden under a bushel," but

* See Chapter XVII.

should be shared with one's fellows, I began to advise and supervise the fasting of others on the same lines. The rest of this book is therefore largely devoted to results obtained on those suffering from a variety of diseases, including medically diagnosed cases of cancer, Bright's disease, gangrene, and many others which from the orthodox standpoint are labelled incurable.

CHAPTER V.

GANGRENE

Gangrene, described in simple language as " death of a part," is regarded as hopeless of cure by the orthodox physician. " Gangrene has set in " is a phrase invariably accepted as the last stage which precedes the almost immediate decease of the victim. Where gangrene sets in after a finger, toe or limb has been amputated, it is often fatal, especially in the case of persons past middle age. All the same, I have proved that gangrene can be easily cured.

My first acquaintance with the ravages of gangrene was in 1891 when I was a schoolboy of ten. My closest schoolmate had complained of face-ache for some days before being taken to a local dentist for the extraction of a tooth far back in the jaw. Unfortunately some of the jaw came away with the molar, and gangrene set in. Drugs and ointments were applied to reduce (or perhaps better said *suppress*) the swelling, and the boy died ten days later.

It so happened that at the same time as my schoolmate was suffering, I also had a swollen cheek. But the remedy my mother applied (she was a farmer's daughter, by the way) was a very different one from the " scientific " ones the doctors had applied to my young friend. True, my own swollen cheek was the result of having been stung by a lot of bees, owing to my having disturbed a colony of those interesting little creatures. All the same it was very painful, till my mother completely cured it by first bathing my face in urine and then binding it up with pieces of linen wrung out in the same healing fluid. My cheek was normal in a few hours.

This treatment was suggested to the parents of my schoolmate with the gangrenous jaw—but merely to be rejected with scorn and expressions of disgust. I have since come to know that urine compresses combined with urine-drinking and fasting could have saved my unfortunate friend.

About a year later a young man of our acquaintance died of either gangrene, medical treatment for the condition, or perhaps both. While he was ill, I used to go and read to him ; and during one of my visits, the doctor called. He was a very loquacious practitioner, and after a few cheering stock phrases, added that whoever found a cure for this dreadful affliction would merit a crown of gold. Had he " read, marked, learned and inwardly digested " the old book I have already quoted, on the value of urine for " *any green wound* " he might have known that a cure had already been found years ago. As it was, I little thought then that it would be given to me to prove the truth of that sentence, and much less did the thought occur to me that it would not be a crown of gold I should receive, but metaphorically speaking, a crown of thorns ! For although the story is not relevant to this book, I have had to suffer for my doctrines and their demonstration.

The first case of gangrene I ever treated was in 1920. The patient was a lady of fifty-three. She had been in the care of a well-known Bradford physician who was an authority on fasting and dietetics. Anaemia had developed, the lungs showed signs of grave disturbance, and there was a gangrenous condition in one foot, with a number of skin eruptions of varying dimensions on each leg. There was also a jaundiced condition which had turned her complexion to that of an Eurasian, and the whites of her eyes yellow. Her abdomen was dis-

32

tended and hard, and her body had become thin and scraggy almost to emaciation.

Although the doctor was quite willing that my method should be tried for at least a month, I was loathe to advise upon the case, for I felt that no period of less than sixty to seventy days would restore the patient to health. However, to my surprise, some encouraging developments occurred fairly quickly, and gave me the first opportunity of observing that gangrene is far from being that hopeless condition which the public and the doctors have been led to believe.

By dint of fasting the patient on her own urine and water, and rubbing urine into her body and applying urine compresses, at the end of ten days the kidneys and bowels were working " overtime," and though the eruptions had increased, they were less irritable. The breathing became normal and easy, the patient slept better, and above all, the gangrenous foot began to show signs of healing.

By the eighteenth day of the fast the foot was quite normal; the urine had formed new skin, and there was no trace whatever of the livid abrasions. The foot had healed without even leaving a scar.

Yet need we be surprised, once we understand that urine is not dead matter, but so to say, flesh, blood and vital tissues in living solution?

As the result of this cure, I was invited to take on another case of gangrene. It was that of a woman in the early forties. Her right leg was in such a state of putrefaction that her medical adviser had urged amputation of the limb.

The trouble had begun nearly two years previously with a swelling at the ankle. This had been ascribed to her occupation which entailed much kneeling on a hard stone floor. She had submitted herself to many treatments, both orthodox and unorthodox, but her afflictions merely increased. She suffered from severe constipation, piles, eczema, anaemia, insomnia, tic nerveux, general depression, sore mouth and tongue, faceache, eruptions at each corner of the lips—and above all, more cavities had occurred in the gangrenous leg. In spite of her tribulations, however, she was a woman of great spirit, and I had no difficulty in persuading her to fast on all the urine she passed, and up to six half-pints a day of *cold* water, which she always *sipped*.

During the first five days of the penance the eruptions began to disappear, and the skin in every part of her body began to look healthier in every respect. The face-ache vanished by the second day, on the third night she slept soundly after weeks of insomnia, and by the end of the first week, the bowels and kidneys were working " overtime " and the piles were cured. In a fortnight there was no sign of the gangrene, and new skin had grown in place of the cavities. The diseased leg, which previously had become twice the size of the other one, was now completely normal—not even a scar remaining anywhere to remind her of what she had suffered ! I subsequently put my recovered patient on an exclusive diet of grapes, bananas and raw tomatoes for a week in small quantities, added fresh unpasteurised milk for the second week, and in the third week finally got her back on a normal diet.

According to my experience, gangrene is often much quicker in response than many other major or " killing " diseases, a matter which may be seen from a few brief case-sheets which I now will add. I should mention that nearly all these cases were treated after the physicians had urged amputation.

Mrs. E. Gangrenous feet and toes following upon paralysis after vaccines had been administered. 48 days fast.   Urine healed feet and toes in the first 20 days.

Mr. D.   Diabetic gangrene of left forearm.   Fasted 48 days for the diabetes.   Arm completely normal after 18 days. No scar.

Mr. J.W.B. (60 years old).   Gangrene of first and second joints of thumb, caused by a hammer-blow in mason work.   Treated for 18 weeks as an out-patient at Leeds G.I.   Bone removed up to first joint.   Discolouration spread towards wrist.   Fasted according to my method, applied urine compresses to whole hand, wrist and arm.   Cured in one week.

Miss C.A. (aged 10 in 1930.)   Anaemia.   Gangrene of both legs following suppressive treatment for psoriasis. Large areas of skinless and livid flesh in both calves. Fasted 18 days.   Cure complete.   No more anaemia, no more psoriasis, no scars from gangrenous legs.   Grew 1½ inches during fast.   Is now a member of the A.T.S. in H.M. Forces.   Height above the average.

Mrs. B.   Gangrenous finger, also severe conjunctivitis following a year's use of atropin.   Fasted 12 days for gangrene, then a week later undertook a second fast for the conjunctivitis which cleared up the 23rd day.   Age 38 in 1927.   Still looks much the same age.

Mr. J.I. (age 54 at the time.)   Thumb cut by fish-bone. Doctor attended him the same day.   Gangrene ensued. Surgeon's decision to amputate rejected.   Fasted 14 days. Body rubbed with urine, finger poulticed in very strong old urine.   Improvement after three days of treatment. Cure complete after twelve days.

Mr. N. (age about 55 at the time.)   Tubercular gangrene of both legs.   Surgeons wanted to amputate the limbs.   His wife refused.   Condition of patient very emaciated.   Great depression after much drugging.

Fasted 42 days according to my method.   Now walks as well as any man, and enjoys the exercise.

Mrs. L. (age 48 at the time.)   Gangrene of both legs and feet after spilling a large vessel of boiling fat over them.   Treated with plasters during three weeks by the physicians.   Result disastrous.   Fasted 28 days, with the usual treatment I advocate.   Marked improvement after ten days.   Return to normal health after a fortnight.

Many other cases could be cited.   But as I do not wish to swell the bulk of this book with an unnecessary number of case-sheets when a few should be sufficient to convince any but the most prejudiced, I will forbear. I think I may say that what I have here put forward should explode the dogma that gangrene is incurable.

We will now provide evidence which should explode another medical dogma—namely the " incurability " of cancer.

CHAPTER VI.

GROWTHS AND CANCER (?)

In 1912 the late Dr. F. Forbes-Ross, of London, a fully qualified physician, wrote a book entitled *Cancer —Its Genesis and Treatment*. He had during twenty-five years of practice come to the conclusion that malignancy and other growths were due to a diet deficient in natural salts—especially in potash. By putting his patients on a more balanced diet (such as I advocate), and administering potash-salts in an assimilable form, he cured a large number of cases of that dread disease. and yet after his death, not one of his colleagues or one single hospital could be induced to take up the treatment —so firmly had the dogma taken hold of the Medical Profession that cancer must be treated exclusively by the knife or radium.   His book is now out of print.   But another book by a Surgeon, Mr. C. P. Childe, advocating speedy interference with the knife the moment a lump looks at all suspicious, is still in print, or was so until quite recently.   (See *Doctors, Disease and Health*, also *Victory over Cancer*, and *Health, Diet and Commonsense*, by Cyril Scott.)

I am not prepared to pronounce on the merits or demerits of Dr. Forbes-Ross's method, for I have not required to try it.   But the treatment of his book shows how little the spirit of democracy prevails in the Medical Profession, and should give intelligent members of the public an inkling as to why cancer is *still* said to be an incurable disease now that the dictum is no longer true . . . if it ever was strictly true.   It would have been more veracious to say that many *patients* suffering from

37

cancer have proved to be incurable. But as I have else-where implied, so have many patients suffering from influenza.

As for surgical treatment of cancerous growth, the late Dr. Rabagliati,* of Bradford, admitted to me that in the earlier part of his career, before I knew him, he had performed no fewer than five hundred major opera-tions for growths, and that it was the uniform lack of success with the knife that had caused him to search for other means of more effectively treating cancer—though unfortunately in vain.

My first case of medically diagnosed cancer was that of a nurse in the late sixties. She had nursed over fifty cases of malignancy in the course of her professional activities, and it says little for the policy of extirpating cancerous growths, that long before she herself developed one, she had vowed that never would she submit to the knife. She was one of many of those in a position to know from the sufferings she had witnessed that however painful a growth may be *before* an operation, the pain is mild in comparison to what is experienced *after* it when the cancer recurs.

When I first saw her, she had had the growth for some months, and it had already extended from both breasts right over both shoulders. It gave her little trouble beyond occasional twinges. She had not con-sulted a doctor about it, but one day, being laid up with influenza, she was obliged to send for a medical man, who, while examining her, discovered the condition of her breast, lamented the fact that it was already too late to operate—and gave her ten days more to live!

The case then came into my hands. A short fast on

* Dr. Rabagliati was well-known in the Medical Profession, and his name occurs in many medical books published both in this country and in U.S.A.

the patient's own urine, plus water, was undertaken. It lasted ten days. Then a light diet was prescribed on the one meal a day plan, along with the free internal use of the urine passed. No effect on the growth was observed ; but the general health and spirits of the patient improved in an astonishing manner. Subsequently the growth itself gave her no further trouble. She retired to a seaside place to live with a relative who scoffed at my theories, and though doctors had failed to cure her of asthma, worshipped at the shrine of medical ortho- doxy. My erstwhile patient died six years later, two hours after a physician had given her some innocent- looking pellets for a cold. I had only seen her once after 1918-19.

This case, from my point of view, was, of course, un- satisfactory. But it serves in some measure to show what many unorthodox physicians have maintained, viz., that if growths are not interfered with by the knife, they do not necessarily kill the patient, and even may cause no trouble.

A case is cited in one of the medical books, relative to an old lady who lived to 96, and had had a cancerous growth of the breast since she was forty ! Various doc- tors she had called in for minor ailments had wished to excise it. but she had always refused on the grounds that it gave her no pain or inconvenience. Moreover she did not believe in the knife.

Since my first " cancer " case, I have treated, in various stages of the disease, a large number of further cases diagnosed as cancerous, and even after some of them had been treated either medically or surgically. In consequence, I have been enabled to collect much interesting data on the subject—most of which conflicts with allopathic theories and popular assumptions. Seeing, however the dogma obtains that genuine cancer is incurable, and seeing that a law has been passed prohibiting any layman even to hint that he can cure (or presumably *has* cured) malignancy, we must assume that all those cases hereafter mentioned which were alleged by the Profession to be cancerous had been wrongly diagnosed.

First I may briefly mention *en masse* the cases of five women I will classify as ABC, because all were unprejudiced by any kind of previous treatment, and every one of them was of recent development. Their cases at least suggest the wisdom of prompt and correct measures. I should stress, however, at the outset, that not one of these patients had been labelled cancer cases. Nevertheless to be on the safe side, I fasted every one of them my way, in addition to applying urine compresses, with complete success ; for in addition to the disappearance of the growths, the treatment resulted in a state of general health far in excess of that experienced prior to the fasts. In fact their growths disappeared so completely that they were all convinced that they could not have been malignant ; especially as I make a point of never employing such terms as cancer, malignancy or even tumour during my consultations. Besides, it must be freely admitted that every lump or nodule that forms on the human body is not a malignant growth—although only a surgeon is credited with the ability or the authority to label it either malignant or otherwise. The ruling unfortunately results in many comparatively harmless lumps being labelled as malignant when such may not be the fact, or it may result in an operation being advised in case they should *become* malignant. Thus, hundreds of trifling lumps have been treated surgically as a major affliction, and cancer has eventually developed, because as yet, neither doctors nor laymen realise that the surest way to invite malignancy is the mutilation of the female breast or other

40

parts of the human body.*

I will now give the case-history of Mrs. R. (1923).
She was in the early forties at the time. Condition—
anaemic, under average height, below normal weight,
lump about the size of a hen's egg in one of her breasts.
Diagnosed as cancer by the late Dr. Rabagliati, and
immediate operation urged, but firmly refused. Fasted
on urine and drank 2½ pints of plain cold tap-water daily.
Her husband rubbed her from head to foot with his own
urine for two hours a day, and packs wrung out in urine
were placed over *both* breasts day and night. *Cure in
ten days.* Returned to Dr. Rabagliati on twelfth day
after last visit to him, and he could find no trace of
abnormality in the breast. Anaemia had vanished also,
and the patient had been restored to perfect health.

Here is another case (1925). Middle-aged woman.
Growth of some proportions situated near the armpit.
Two surgeons advised operation, but made a concession
to her daughter's suggestion that the patient might rest
and take very light nourishment before facing the ordeal.
The operation was accordingly arranged to take place in
the hospital a week hence. However, as the patient's
daughter had derived much benefit herself from urine-
fasting, she prevailed on her mother to try the treatment
in the interim. *In five days not a trace of the growth
was left.* I may add that two -days after the patient
should have presented . herself at the hospital for the
operation, the family doctor called in. He was indig-
nant at having his advice and arrangements flouted
in this "independent" manner; but when having
thoroughly examined the patient he found her condition

* For instance, San Francisco is a surgically ridden city; it has
few physicians but hundreds of surgeons. Therefore we are
not astonished when we read that "the mortality from
cancer in San Francisco exceeds that of any other American
city." (See *Victory over Cancer* by Cyril Scott.)

41

entirely normal, there was nothing more to be said. Subsequently he called in his colleagues, who, to express it mildly, were extremely astonished, and being human, were not altogether pleased. I merely add this part of the story to show that the patient had been properly examined after her recovery. She is at the time of writing many years older, and quite well.

A case may now be cited relative to a youngish woman who had developed a growth in her breast. I cite it because the trouble disappeared in the shortest period I had yet witnessed for what might have been a malignant tumour or merely a swollen milk-gland. I think, none the less, that had the patient put herself in the hands of physicians, they would have advised an operation just as they have done in hundreds of similar cases. On seeing her, I at once advocated a fast on her own urine, plus tap-water, and urine compresses—in short, the usual procedure I advise. *At the end of four days the growth had entirely disappeared.*

And now I will mention the case of a lady who came to me in 1927. It is instructive as showing once again that operations merely deal with effects and do not remove the *cause* of the disease from the body. The lady in question was 45, over stout, and had a growth of some size in her left breast, *the right one having been removed two years previously for a similar growth.* She fasted and was treated according to my method for nineteen days, and then reported that the growth had entirely vanished. As she was still too fleshy, I advised her to continue the fast. On the 28th day, I examined her, to find no trace of the lump, and to see a woman looking much younger and far less matronly in figure.

The following case shows that one and the same methods may result in curing complaints which have no apparent connection with each other. A young lady came to me with a swollen right breast, near the centre of which was a nasty, suspicious-looking lump. There were also two large ulcers under the arm-pit. She had been invited by the family doctor to enter the hospital for observation, but declined, seeing that her mother had accepted a similar invitation, had been operated upon—and subsequently buried. Moreover she herself, having suffered from chronic peritonitis, had had her appendix excised, but without curing the peritonitis. She started by fasting four days on my system, but had to break the fast to satisfy her insistent relatives. Nevertheless, after three days she resumed the fast, and the second time fasted for nineteen days. Already after the tenth day there was a marked improvement, and at the end of the nineteen days no trace was left of the lump on her breast or the ulcers in her arm-pit. There was not even a scar. But the peritonitis had not cleared up (perhaps because of scarred tissue resulting from the operation on appendix) and so a little later she fasted for thirty-five days. This had the desired effect.

These case-sheets should serve to show that Nature is a far more efficient Healer than are so-termed scientific methods which involve mutilation. If people who observe suspicious lumps on their bodies would only resort to these natural methods I have outlined, and resort to them at once, Nature would not fail them. But those who wait till the eleventh hour may have to pay the penalty for their procrastination.

All the same, I think the dogma anent the fatality of cancer will die hard, because as soon as a case is cured by whatever methods, the tendency is to assert : " Then it couldn't have been cancer." Doctors who resort to this phrase forget that it is a poor reflection on the diagnostic powers of the orthodox physician or surgeon. Moreover what are we to make of the following admission by the authors of *The Breast* in which book Drs. Dearer and

Macfarland wrote: "I have operated on some thousand cases of cancer, and they all returned but six, and *they* were not cancer"? And again: "The acknowledged poor results obtained by surgery in any sort of cancer *are well known to the profession.*" (Dr. G. E. Ward, Howard Kelley Hospital. Baltimore. Italics mine.) Yet if these poor results are so well known, then why does the profession continue to advocate the knife, and ignore those who obtain good results without surgery, as did Dr. Forbes-Ross and others since his death? Mention may be made here of Dr. W. F. Koch, of Detroit, who, over a period of 20 years, has cured hundreds of cases of cancer, both external and internal, by a subtle chemical formula. Yet far from being recognised by the Orthodox Cancer Ring in U.S.A., he has been scoffed at and even persecuted. Why should this be so?

I leave the intelligent reader to draw his own conclusions, and will proceed to cite one or two cases where the doctors, although advocating the knife, held out very poor prospects of recóvery, if indeed any at all. These cases include growths in other sites of the body, as hitherto I have only mentioned breast cases. The reader now being familiar with the treatment, I will merely give the barest details.

Young man, 28, in 1920. Given three days to live. Condition variously diagnosed as either cancer of the gullet or venereal disease. Complete cure. Patient still alive.

Lady of 62; diagnosed cancer of the bowel. Colotomy advised by the profession, but refused. Was under 6 stone and rapidly wasting away. Cured in three weeks. At the date of writing is 84.

Lady of 42; diagnosed cancer of breast. Excision advised, to be followed by strict regime; but only faint

44

hope of a cure offered by the profession.   Patient refused
operation.   Complete cure by the fasting-urine method.
Is still alive and well after 21 years.

Lady of 40.   In 1935 developed the type of growth
sometimes called " rope cancer."   Surgeons pressed for
immediate excision but offered no hope of a permanent
cure, saying that return and spread of growth practically
inevitable.   Cured by the urine-fast, etc., in twenty-three
days.   Is not only still well, but looks young and beautiful.

It may be of interest to the reader if I cite what the
late Dr. Rabagliati—that frank, enlightened and broad-
minded physician — said relative to the treatment of
diagnosed cancer and growths by the methods I have
outlined.

" I have examined women with what would in
orthodox care have resulted in the removal of one
or both breasts.   These happy mortals have declined
my advice, gone under urine-therapy and returned to
my consulting rooms without even a scar to suggest
the healing of ' incurable malignancy.'

" Many of these females have found the lump or
lumps to disappear within a fortnight, some in as
few as four days ; all of which suggests that Mr.
Armstrong is probably correct in his suggestion that
most lumps are not malignant until *after* surgical
and drug interference, and that in the incipient
stages, the so-called King of Terrors . . . is a very
ordinary affair when tackled promptly . . . in the
right way—the way of breaking down boils, ulcers,
tumours and cancers into the blood-stream . . .

" If, however, any layman claimed and produced
a thousand cured cases on one platform, I doubt
if it would impress my profession—even claims for
the improvement of cancer victims are either openly

ridiculed or ignored.   It is a sad reflection that my profession thrives on disease and the inhuman propaganda of official scaremongering and the promise of to-morrow, some other day, or *never,* for the diseases my profession and others have so long exploited."

Some Prevailing Theories as to Cancer Causation, etc.

To relieve the monotony of an uninterrupted recital of case-histories in this book, we may give a few moments' attention to various theories as to the causes of cancer, in order to see if they have any bearing on my thesis.

Because cancer occurs less frequently among vegetarians, some enthusiastic non meat-eaters declare that the consumption of meat is the prime cause of malignancy. But if this were true, then all persons except vegetarians (unless they died before the age when cancer is usually said to develop) would, without exception, succumb to its ravages.   Moreover some non meat-eaters have and do die of cancer.   " Well, at any rate," rejoin the vegetarians, " meat-eating favours disease in the human body, and as Sir Arbuthnot Lane maintained, cancer cannot develop in a healthy organism.   If a man who has been for a long time a vegetarian suddenly starts to eat meat, disturbances ensue.   The case may be quoted of a vegetarian who averred that there must be some animal fat in a certain brand of rather unusual-tasting biscuits, because whenever he had consumed one, he noticed that there followed a slight attack of fever." Maybe ; but as against that, I could quote the case of a young man who, having over a long period lived on a diet which included meat but excluded pastries and chocolates, developed boils and a skin eruption as soon as he ate those aliments. From this I might agree, if so minded, that as pastries and chocolates produced these disturbances and favoured disease, they were the cause

46

of cancer ! Just as at one time some people believed that tomatoes were its cause.

The truth is that wishful thinking has played as much part in the question of malignancy as it has in other vexed questions. Vegetarians want to believe that meat-eating " is the root of all evil " and so pounce upon it as the cause of malignancy and a host of other ailments. But if we bring commonsense into the matter another explanation appears to be far more reasonable. Sensible vegetarians live on a less de-natured diet than do the generality of meat-eaters and hence are less likely to develop cancer. On the other hand, those " unscientific " vegetarians who live mostly on macaroni, starch-foods, boiled instead of steamed vegetables, and on pastries, puddings. etc., made of white flour, are living as much on a de-natured diet as any person who subsists to a large extent on such rubbishy aliments plus meat—very often tinned at that.

The cause of cancer must be obvious to those who " become as little children " and do not blind themselves to truth by the blinkers of pseudo scientific learning, and thus overlook the *simple* because so pre-occupied with the *complex*. Even so, some of them are obliged to fall back on the simple in the end. After writing an enormous tome overloaded with the conflicting theories and dogmatical pronouncements of cancer researchers both orthodox and unorthodox, Prof. F. L. Hoffman (of U.S.A.) comes to the startling (!) conclusion that, after all, food may have something to do with the incidence of cancer !

And yet, granted this to be the case, in most instances it is not the food which people consume that is its cause, but the deficiency, as already implied, of those essential mineral salts to be found in the foods which they do *not* consume, but ought to consume in order to keep the blood and tissues in a healthy condition.

I am aware that of late the discovery has been made (*not* by the Cancer Ring) that some people who have lived for a length of time in a house situated over an underground stream, have eventually developed cancer— an observation which may account for so-termed " cancer houses "—but we have still to discover whether such people would have developed the dread disease if they had lived on a well-balanced diet. It would be also instructive to discover whether those cases of " spontaneous " disappearance of cancerous growths have followed upon removing to another place of dwelling. Of such cases the well-known surgeon, Mr. Hastings Gilford, wrote (in 1925) the significant words : " Though cancer is commonly regarded as inevitably fatal, many cases are recorded of its ' spontaneous ' disappearance—and nothing can be more certain than that these recorded cases are very few in comparison with those which are left unrecorded. " (!) A damaging admission, by the way, which suggests, as Mr. Ellis Barker and others have already suggested, that the Medical Profession and the Cancer Ring may be anxious to keep the real truth about malignancy from the lay public.

One more theory may be here cited, viz., that the excessive use of common salt (which is *not* a food) is conducive to cancer. According to *" The Biochemic System of Medicine "* there are at least twelve important mineral salts which are present in healthy blood and tissues. Why, therefore, take *one* of these salts and administer it in the crude form that Nature never intended, and in quantities in which it does not exist in natural foods? Moreover, if cancer is a fungoid growth, as it has been maintained, then surely a warning may be derived from the fact that gardeners water mushroom beds with warm salt and water solutions with the object of producing a profuse crop. Another suggestive point is that, in spite of eating large quantities of salt in its crude form, the tissues of people who live on an ill-balanced or de-natured diet, can nevertheless register deficiency of sodium chloride (common salt). Sodium chloride is necessary—and hence, of course harmless—to the tissues in such minute quantities as are to be found in vegetables, salads, etc., but is harmful when taken into the body as a condiment. The same is relatively true of iron; phosphate of iron being one of the 12 tissue salts. Yet whereas practitioners of the *Biochemic System of Medicine* frequently cure anaemia by giving infinitesimal doses of ferrum phosphate, the allopath, by giving it in far too large doses, merely upsets the patient's digestion and fails to cure the trouble.

All this again points to the simple truth that all diseases from anaemia to cancer, provided they are not produced by some structual alteration or some deep-seated psychological cause, have their origin in wrong feeding.

As to how far fear-thoughts are conducive to cancer, it would be hard to determine. But in any case fear is an unpleasant emotion as well as being a harmful one if long protracted. Yet unfortunately the Medical Profession by their methods of advertising, foster the very thing they should be the first to alleviate, as Dr. Marie Stopes implied in a letter to *The Yorkshire Post*, August 4, 1938. Referring to the report of a speech by Lord Horder on quack medicines, she wrote :—

" As I do not use such medicines but believe in British fair play, I ask your readers to consider that (a) Lord Horder objected primarily to the ' fear ' created by quack advertising : but surely all such minor fears put together are not so serious as the fear of cancer, entirely created by the medical profession, the advertising of which is in their their hands and that of the recognised hospitals; (b) that all quack medicines are only swallowed and rubbed on and cannot do a fraction of the frightful injury to our race done by the medical profession's injections into the bloodstream and tissues of active virus, dirt and anti-toxins. Lord Horder objects to 'unscrupulous advertising,' but the most unscrupulous piece of advertising I have ever seen was recently put out by the medical profession itself urging that foul poison, pasteurised milk, on the public.

"It is surely clear that Lord Horder's speech was a superb example of the pot calling the kettle black."

This letter speaks for itself. And *apropos* of quacks, a real quack in the worst sense of the word is the man who professes to cure what he knows he cannot cure. Before it became illegal for me to treat cancer, I never once professed to cure anyone after he or she had been subjected to radium treatment. Cancer itself was child's play to deal with in comparison to the after-effects of radium, and had I offered any hope of curing these I should have been a quack imposter of the most bare-faced type.

CHAPTER VII.

BRIGHT'S DISEASE: CASE HISTORIES

Bright's disease is defined as "a morbid condition of the kidneys"; the term is "generic," and includes several forms of acute and chronic disease of the kidney, usually associated with albumen in the urine, and frequently with dropsy, and with various secondary symptoms. Its causes are said to be "the effects of fever, especially scarlet fever, exposure to wet and cold, as a contributory cause only, the action of irritating drugs, alcohol, etc. Dr. G. Johnson found, by an analysis of 200 cases, that intoxicating drinks cause 29 per cent. of all cases, and 12 per cent. arise from scarlet fever." (Dr. E. Harris Ruddock, M.D., *Vade Mecum*).

According to *The Biochemic System of Medicine* (G. W. Carey, M.D., of U.S.A.) Bright's disease is primarily caused by a lack of phosphate of calcium in the body. He writes: "When the phosphate of lime molecules fall below the standard of quantity, the albumen with which they are associated is, of course, thrown out of circulation, and if this albumen reaches the outer world by the kidney route, a case of albuminuria is developed."

According to the practitioners of this System, the chief remedy therefore is phosphate of lime, administered in infinitesimal doses as Nature would supply it in such foods as are not de-natured by refining processes. In other words, Bright's disease is caused by deficiency diet, viz., a diet lacking in the essential mineral salts to keep the blood and tissues healthy. To quote Dr. Carey again, "Biochemists have clearly demonstrated the fact that when a deficiency of the cell-salts of the blood occurs, the organic matter with which those salts have been associated is thrown out of the vital circulation." It is worthy of note that although the *Biochemic System of Medicine* claims to be able to cure deficiency diseases, it stresses the fact that it cannot cure the effects of gourmandising.

The incidence of Bright's disease dates back to early times, but it considerably increased during last century and onwards, and in its worst forms has been the cause of many untimely deaths.

It is a singular fact that during the first three years of my career as a urine-therapist, although I had contacted many cases of cancer, diabetes, consumption and valvular disease of the heart, not once until 1920 was I confronted with a genuine case of the disease, of which dropsy is but a symptom. (Dropsy occurs in diseases other than Bright's disease.)

My first case was one of the most testing I have since experienced. Here are the particulars:

Mrs. C. Age, in the early forties. Given two days to live by the doctors. Breathing somewhat difficult. Urine very scanty, thick and looking like a mixture of blood and pus. She had been a very fine specimen of womanhood, judging from photographs taken a year or so previously. Her normal weight for a woman of her height had been 144lbs., but when I was first called in to see her she weighed roughly 280lbs. (20 stone). In spite of the doctor's verdict, however, I did not think that she looked like a dying woman, though, to say the least her condition was a very serious and painful one. Fortunately for the case, she had two elderly and humane nurses who had little faith, notwithstanding their profession, in drug and medical treatment. Of these two women I can never speak highly enough and of the broad-minded manner in which they gave me their full co-operation. Judging from the contents of the medicine table, it was hardly to be wondered at that they had lost faith in drugs, for there was such an array of bottles that my indignation was aroused by the way the unfortunate patient had been "experimented on." Nevertheless on the strength of what I had seen in far worse local conditions of heart affections, breathing difficulties, stasis, etc., I promised her speedy relief from her most distressing symptoms, and predicted that she would find her ability to void urine increase at least a hundredfold within one week; so powerful is the effect of drinking one's *own* urine, which serves to break up congestions in every part of the body.

My prediction came true. Within four days the flow of urine had increased from a bare 2oz. (it was very high in aroma, hot, thick, cloudy and full of casts) to about 200ozs. in twenty-four hours. Moreover it began to change into a much clearer and far more freely expressed liquid, gradually approaching the appearance of rainwater. By the fourth day after drinking every drop she passed, it was practically tasteless, free from odour, and in no sense of the word objectionable.

In addition to the urine, Mrs. C. was permitted to take, by sipping it, as much tap-water as she desired—this amounted to about 108ozs. in the twenty-four hours; although I should add that after the third day, thirst had become well-nigh absent.

From the fourth day onward, I had lost all anxiety about the case, and except for short infrequent visits, left the treatment in the hands of the two intelligent and helpful nurses.

By the twenty-third day the patient was showing such signs of complete recovery that one of the nurses begged

53

me to try the effect of a little grated raw carrot juice flavoured with lemon. The result was a set-back. Within two hours, a rash covering a considerable area and attended with much irritation appeared on each arm. At the same time the flow of urine was impeded and there was much swelling and irritation in the abdomen. Cloths soaked in one of the nurse's urine were placed over the abdominal region, whilst both arms were gently rubbed and bathed with the same fluid. After four hours the abdomen absorbed the moisture from the urine-packs, and the flow of urine re-commenced. This was taken internally, and the following day, except for the rash and irritation, the patient's condition was the same as before the carrot had been eaten. As for the rash, it took nearly a week before it vanished.

One of the features of urine-therapy is the rubbing of the patient's whole body with urine at given intervals for two hours at a stretch; that is, provided the patient is not too weak and emaciated to stand it. Mrs. C. was therefore rubbed twice a day for two hours with one or other of the nurses' urine. By the 48th day, the patient had so far become normal, that on the 49th day we broke her fast by giving her the juice of an orange at noon, and a whole orange to suck at 4 p.m. That same day she voided and took urine freely—which meant that all was now in order. At 6.30 she was given a small piece of steamed fish and two steamed potatoes in their jackets. She weighed now 119lbs. Next day she had two small meals, which she was advised to fletcherise, i.e., chew to pulp before swallowing. In a week she was on her feet, dressed in her clothes of the previous year, and able to walk easily from room to room.

Although recovered, she kept up the practice of taking her own urine, as also rubbing it into the body (the most important areas are the face and the neck) with astonishing results on the skin, hair, complexion, and her general appearance. Indeed, urine is the skin food *par excellence* as also the remedy for every kind of skin disease.

And here ends the long case-history of Mrs. C. who was given " only two days to live "! Incidentally, both her husband and the two nurses became strong converts to urine-therapy, and I may add, to a well-balanced, as opposed to a de-natured, diet.

Mrs. C's, case attracted much attention as far as the lay public was concerned, but not, as I then innocently hoped, from the medical fraternity. For, as Dr. Freud, the discoverer of Psycho-analysis, has pointed out, no matter what evidence, many people only allow themselves to believe what they *wish* to believe, and likewise they disbelieve what they wish to disbelieve. All the same, there are extenuating circumstances where the medical profession is concerned. Until a lot more "spade work" has been done to put an end to prudery, the chances are that if a doctor told his patients to fast and drink their own urine, he would merely be regarded as mad or disgusting, and the patients would immediately seek the advice of some other physician. Besides, why do most people seek medical advice? In order to be told how to counteract the effects of their self-indulgencies. If one doctor tells them they must give up this and that, they then go to another doctor who tells them they need not give up this or that; and being delighted with his advice, follow it—very often to their own undoing.

Enough said—Mrs. C's case was instrumental in bringing the case of Mr. B. whose condition had also been diagnosed as Bright's disease. Mr. B. had for years subsisted on the usual ill-balanced deficiency diet, rendered even more deficient by non-conservative cooking, and rendered more "tasty " by the adjunct of condiments. He was not a big eater, but he drank some eight cups of tea a day and smoked about twenty-five cigarettes on an average. When he came to me in 1920, he had been under two doctors for some time, during which period his weight had increased from 280lbs. to 420lbs. Like Mrs. C., he had finally been given two days to live.

In June, 1920, he began a fast which lasted 49 days. By the fourth day of his penance he was passing water as clear and as tasteless almost as rain-water, and his swellings began to vanish with astonishing rapidity. He had been anaemic, but at the end of the seven weeks, his anaemia had disappeared. His weight was now 105lbs., and he looked in every respect as young as he had done 20 years before. (As his photographs showed.)

Mr. B. broke his fast in much the same way as Mrs. C. had done, and like her, became a convert to urine-therapy and a properly balanced, if frugal, diet, viz., he gave up de-natured food and continued to drink his own urine daily, with most gratifying results.

In the same year, more cases came into my hands. Mr. W. (75 at the time), Mrs. L. (38), Mr. B. (55) and also a boy of 11. Each case presented features worthy of recital at length, but brevity must suffice. Mr. W., in spite of his age, fasted 53 days—which serves to show that age is no obstacle. Mrs. L. 42 days, Mr. B. 60 days. In the case of the boy, a fortnight proved sufficient to effect a cure. All the cases were attended with the same happy ending as that of Mrs. C. And here let me add that the policy of forcing sick people to eat " in order to keep up their strength " is in my opinion responsible for thousands of untimely deaths. Food cannot be assimilated by a sick body which is already full of obstructive matter. The only " food " for sick people is urine, seeing that among its other functions it replaces tissue in a manner nothing else can do. As for drugs, many of those poisonous ones employed have serious cumulative effects for which there are no antidotes.

After 1920, during the next two years, I had over thirty cases of Bright's disease and other affections of the bladder and kidneys to advise upon, and in no instance did it take longer than from four to fourteen days on urine fasts to restore normality, and a satisfactory state of general health. These cases having yielded to treatment so much more readily than the ones aforesighted, I classified them in my notes as A.B.C. cases.

I will briefly cite one more of the serious cases. Man of 60, after two years' constant medical supervision and treatment for heart, developed Bright's disease. Finally, given up by his two doctors, specialist was called in. He saw the victim at the stage when his eyes were starting from his head, tongue was dreadfully swollen and protruding from mouth, whilst his lips were three times their normal size. Specialist said the case was hopeless. Nothing more to be done. I undertook the case. Patient passed 40 pints of water five days later, and returned to business in six weeks—cured.

CHAPTER VIII.

A Case of Leucocythaemia or Leukaemia
(Splenic Anaemia)

That remarkable naturopath, the late Louis Kuhne, of Leipsic, declared that disease was a unity, and with trifling variations should be always treated in the same way. He maintained that all diseases, no matter what their names or sites, invariably rise from the same cause, viz., an encumbrance of foreign matter in the body. He said it was absurd to treat an organ separately (as specialists often do) for, as goes without saying, any organ or limb is a part of the body, and to think to cure an eye, an arm, a leg or what-not merely by treating it locally is the height of pseudo scientific folly! If an eye is diseased, there is something in the body itself which is causing that disease. For instance, he gives the case of a woman who was going blind. He treated her whole body, ridding it of its " cloggings, " and the eye-trouble cleared up automatically. She had suffered for years from bleeding piles; the orthodox physicians, having finally operated on her. Soon afterwards she started to lose her sight. The safety-valve had been blocked up by this measure, the operation, declared Kuhne, and the poisons went to her eyes. (See *The New Science of Healing.*)

Kuhne effected many remarkable cures by his method, but would have effected even a greater number had he known the value of urine as a means of replacing wasted tissue. Yet he was right when he declared that all diseases (except those caused by traumatism or structual defects) could be cured by one means, as I myself have

58

demonstrated. The *name* of the disease is of merely academic interest, and has nothing to do with the curing of it. All the same, for the sake of convenience, and to prove this fact, I have advisedly specified the diseases treated, and will now give the case-sheets relative to what is termed Leucocythaemia or Leukaemia.

The patient, Mr. P.C., was brought in a taxi to my house by two of my "disciples." He was too ill to walk into my room unsupported, looked very pale and wretched, and altogether was obviously in a very bad state. His age was 48, he had lost 4 stone in one year, and another stone during some weeks of medical treatment.

After I had examined him, I said in effect: " Mr. P.C., your condition is medically tabulated as leucocythaemia or splenic anaemia, and according to the Medical Profession, you have but three months to live. Your disease has been brought about by an ill balanced, denatured diet. None the less you can be saved by fasting and urine-therapy. " I went on to explain the details. Then he told me his story. The gist of it was as follows:

Shortly before Easter of that year (1927) he had developed a cold, for which he had " doctored " himself. By the Good Friday, his condition had been such that his wife and his brother had become alarmed and sent for a young physician who had diagnosed high blood-pressure. On a second examination the following day, however, he had said it was not high blood-pressure after all, and that he had found traces of other symptoms, which he did not particularise. A specialist was then called in. He examined the patient, pointed out the region of the swollen spleen to the general practitioner— and diagnosed the case as leucocythaemia. Mr. P.C. was then informed that the disease was rare in England,

and asked if he had ever been to the East or the Tropics? His relatives were told that the malady always proved fatal, but that the patient might live from three to six months if given deep X-ray treatment, drugs, and a series of injections. (No mention was made of diet, except that liver would be good for the patient.) Mr. P.C. accordingly attended at the local infirmary, where he was examined at various times by the visiting physicians, who became interested in him as " a somewhat rare specimen. " All of them were unanimous as to the name of the disease and the length of time the patient had still to live. His blood was tested by the staff pathologist and registered at 556,000 more white corpuscles than red ones per cubic millimeter.

That was the position when Mr. P.C. was brought to me, five weeks after the disease had been given its polysyllabic and high-sounding name.

Mr. P.C. was not an easy patient, and was not prepared to fast without interruption as long a period as I considered essential for his grave condition, which had been complicated by all the medical X-ray treatment he had undergone. However, although he only fasted a week, during which he was rubbed with urine by his wife and friends for lengthy periods (and, of course, he did not omit the essential part of the treatment, the drinking of his own urine), he was so far improved that he could walk into my house unaided. Indeed, his improvement was so marked that, under pressure, I consented to his breaking his fast, provided that I should dictate what and when he should eat, and that the rubbings and the intake of his urine were not discontinued. His food during the next week was to consist of fresh raw fruits (apples, oranges and bananas, chiefly), salads, tomatoes, *steamed* vegetables, potatoes in their jackets, fresh uncooked, unpasteurised milk, and honey; all of which were to be consumed in small quantities. Later on he was permitted steamed fish, meat, etc., in short a well-balanced diet minus tinned meats or twice cooked meats of any sort. He was to continue to drink his own urine. All this he faithfully carried out.

Six weeks from the day I first saw him, Mr. P.C. had a further blood test. This revealed that, whereas the blood count had previously been 556,000 white corpuscles in excess of red, it now showed less than half that amount per cubic millimeter. Mr. P.C. was so cheered by this report that he consented to further fasts of a week's duration. Thus, during the next six weeks he underwent fasts of seven days each. The third and final blood test revealed that the blood content was quite normal. Soon after the twelve weeks in all of vigorous treatment were ended, Mr. P.C. was back at work—a well man.

Nevertheless, the story has no happy ending. Despite my having impressed upon him that his condition had arisen through an ill-balanced " rubbishy " diet, in the course of time (as I afterwards learned) he reverted to his old habits of eating just any " mess " he "fancied. " Although, for two years after his penance and while he kept up rational feeding, he did not even have one cold to contend with, after those two years he gradually began to backslide, and although he had a few boils and colds by the way of warnings, he paid no attention, and finally died during drug treatment for influenza six years after his recovery from his grievous illness.

Truly, " the way of the transgressor is hard. "

Apropos of Mr. P.C.'s case, I was destined to lose an old school friend through the same fatal medical treatment for splenic anaemia. He had for some time been undergoing deep X-ray for this disease, and, learning of my success with Mr. P.C., had resolved to undergo the fasting and urine cure. But it was too late. He died in his own house attended to the last by well-meaning, but alas, deluded professors of the healing art, who thought that science was mightier than Nature!

CHAPTER IX.

Heart Disease : Cases

Although, as Mr. Ellis Barker encouragingly writes, patients with valvular disease of the heart can, with care and a well-balanced diet, live even till 90, yet the disease as such is said to be incurable. Nevertheless, by means of urine-therapy this distressing condition can be completely cured. The following case-history is instructive.

Mr. P. (middle-aged). He had not only been under the doctor for a year suffering from valvular disease of the heart, but was about to undergo an exploratory operation for a suspicious lump in the region of the solar plexus. Very often he had fainted in the street and had been carried into the nearest chemist shop, where he had been fortified by drug tablets which he always carried in his pocket. On his clothing was a tab instructing people what to do when he was overtaken by an attack. Latterly he had suffered from these attacks so frequently, that he came to be known in the vicinity as " Poor Mr. P. " He had been placed on a regime which consisted of his only being allowed one meal per day for five days of the week, whilst over week-ends he was ordered to fast on water only. No exercise was permitted except a short, gentle walk. Smoking was prohibited, and as for medicaments, he was only to have the drug-tablets during an actual attack.

Such was the position when he came into my hands.

The first thing I urged him to do was to drink the urine he passed. As I expected, this proved to be very odorous and turgid at first, but soon cleared up. I instructed Mr. P. how to rub his body with urine, and

63

then rubbed him for about two hours with my own. *En passant*, I may remark that the most important parts of the body to rub are the face, neck and feet. After the rubbing, Mr. P. was washed down with plain, warm tap-water. The following day the treatment was continued for some hours. Subsequently Mr. P. came to my house every morning to be rubbed in the same manner. He did not enter the Nursing Home for observation or the exploratory operation. With regard to food, he was allowed to eat once a day, but only such foods as I advocated. After one month of treatment, he was so far improved that he was able to return to business. In twelve weeks he registered complete health, and no sign either of the valvular disease of the heart or the suspicious lump in the solar plexus remained; a fact which his doctor cheerfully and ungrudgingly admitted. Not once since the day Mr. P. began the treatment did he have a heart attack, and so little did he fear a recurrence that he consigned his drug tablets to the flames!

Should it be supposed that I am the only one who practises urine-therapy with success, the following case-history will serve to contravene the assumption.

Mr. R. Heart disease with dropsy. Feet, legs and abdomen greatly swollen. Heart much dilated. Doctor took a very serious view of the case, and gave the patient only a month to live. He was then induced to try treatment in a well-known Naturopathic Establishment. The treatment, however, proved so unsuccessful and the patient was in such a critical condition that he was requested to leave; seeing that he was expected to die within a fortnight. Mr. R. then heard of the courageous Naturopath, Mr. Oliver Warnock-Fielden, of Harrow who eventually cured him with urine-therapy in six weeks. During the fast his weight was reduced from about 12 to 7 stone 11½lbs. Mr. R. had been a very excessive smoker, and contrary to instructions, smoked to a certain extent during the fast—a matter which somewhat delayed progress. Needless to say, his doctor was very surprised at his cure; the more so as Mr. R. had thought it wise not to divulge *the modus operandi*. As things stand at present, many people who do something so unconventional as to drink their own urine are afraid to be ostracised by society. Their fears are quite understandable, but obstructive to the spread of urine-therapy as a means of helping suffering humanity.

I may here add a word to this chapter relative to what has been pronounced to be one of the causes of heart disease in modern times, viz., serums and vaccines. According to Dr. Benchetrit these measures " are principally responsible for the increase of these two really dangerous diseases, cancer and heart disease. " The doctor adds: " I have been for a long time a serologist and I know what I am talking about. " Dr. Benchetrit is by no means the only doctor to criticise the practice of employing harmful preventatives (or alleged to be preventatives) against acute infectious disease. Dr. S. S. Goldwater, New York Commissioner of Hospitals, pointed out in *The Modern Hospital Magazine* that measures used to check contagious diseases may permit of longer (?) life but not of stronger life. " Chronic diseases, " he adds, " are growing at such a rate that America may become a nation of invalids. More than half the hospital-beds in the United States to-day are occupied by sufferers from chronic mental and physical diseases. Middle-aged and elderly persons are not the only sufferers; many children are victims. " (See *Health Practitioners Journal*, June, 1944.)

One may ask, if sera and vaccines are liable eventually to produce heart-disease and other chronic serious ailments, why then are they boosted by the B.M.A.? For, first of all, as Dr. Alfred Pulford, M.D., has tersely remarked: " Any one who can prevent an occurrence positively that he does not know is bound to occur is indeed a seventh day wonder"; and secondly certain renowned bigwigs in the Medical Profession have demonstrated that the most "deadly" germs are harmless in a healthy body. We read that "Prof. Metchnikoff said he found the bacilli of Asiatic cholera in the waters of many localities, but no epidemic or plague or disease was ever known to be at any of these places before or after his findings . . . . Prof. Tentenkoffer swallowed several million germs of the deadly (?) Asiatic cholera . . . . Nothing happened. To verify the test, Prof. Emmrich made a culture from the intestines of newly dead victims of the disease, and swallowed millions of germs, with no noticeable results! To test even more thoroughly, and in far more frightful conditions, Dr. Thomas Powell allowed the germs of seven deadly (?) diseases to be shot into his blood-stream—and was as alive ten years later as on that day, and as healthy." (Extract from *Naturopath and Herald of Health*.) Nevertheless these facts are not made known to the general public, nor do those who urge members of the community to be immunized against this or that disease inform them that not all doctors are in favour of such measures, being of the opinion that vaccines and serums may later on produce chronic afflictions, not the least of which is heart disease.

CHAPTER X.

FEVERS: MALARIA AND OTHERS

Case of a mysterious fever, which occurs in Africa but is rare in England.

Patient, young lady of 17. Mysteriously stricken. Very weak. Temperature 105. M.D. called in said if recovery took place at all, the victim would be ill for six months and then would be nine months convalescent. Patient's father—a believer in urine-therapy—sent for me. At first I found the victim difficult to deal with, but she finally consented to a urine-fast plus plain water. On the sixth day after she had been stricken, her temperature was still 105, and she was growing rapidly emaciated, her urine being thick, foul and concentrated. But twenty-four hours after starting my treatment the temperature had dropped to 101 and the urine was clearer. In three days the temperature was down to 97, and in five days to 95. Patient bright and lively—all was going well. Doctor much puzzled. Fast was broken at the end of 18 days. The patient's skin was as clear as that of a child. Within a few days of breaking the fast she was up and doing and feeling perfectly well. She continued the use of her own urine and has thrived upon it. Some sixteen years ago she married, and had three children in the first ten years.

Malaria.

This in an infectious disease characterised by paroxysms of intermittent fever, each consisting of a cold, a hot and a perspiring stage. Between the paroxysms the victim appears comparatively well. According to *Materia Medica* all forms of malaria are due to parasites living in the blood. Mosquitoes are infected by sucking human blood.

and in turn infect human beings by biting them. The troublesome and distressing feature of malaria—which the allopaths treat (suppress) with quinine—is that when once contracted it occurs again and again, for under the usual orthodox treatment it merely goes into latency instead of being totally eradicated. Under urine-therapy, however, it is cured once and for all. So far I have never had a case which did not clear up in 10 days or less by dint of fasting on urine and plain water.

Mr. Q. Athletic type. Very temperate and a small eater. Contracted malaria out East. Had it for three years. During the year before I saw him in 1920 had suffered from thirty-six attacks. He dosed himself regularly with quinine. Finally cured himself completely with a urine-fast lasting ten days. No more quinine. Has never had another attack, and has kept in fine health by adhering to his temperate habits and freely partaking of the " water of life. "

Blackwater Fever.

Case related to me by the erstwhile victim. Army man (Major) found by natives in the backwoods to be in a state of delirium due to blackwater fever. They cured him by fasting him for 10 days, by the applying of packs and by inducing him to take his own urine, and plain water. I mention this to stress that I am not the discoverer of urine-therapy.

In this chapter I have limited myself to reciting only one case history of the various fevers mentioned, merely because to do otherwise would be to enlarge the bulk of this book to unwieldly proportions. I will now conclude with some remarks about fever in general, and acute diseases attended with fever.

When doctors try to bring down a patient's temperature by unnatural means, they are frustrating Nature and may be endangering the patient's life, or at best laying up seeds for future troubles. A fever is really a curative process on the part of Nature to burn up certain toxins in the body. Oh yes, we hear of the "miraculous" temperature-reducing effects of wonder drugs for pneumonia, but we do not hear so much of the many people who die of heart-trouble after the fever has been thus miraculously cured! Experience has taught me that there is only one safe way to treat a fever, which, being a curative process, is neither incurable nor need prove fatal if rightly handled. The modus operandi will by now have become so familiar to the reader that it need not be repeated here. I need merely say that not only have I never seen a failure with the urine-fast plus tap water therapy (all the urine passed should be drunk) but that the fall of temperature has taken place within any time from 36 to 72 hours, followed by complete recovery within a few days.

As to why the urine is so thick, foul and scanty in cases of fever, that is not the result of the fever itself but of the condition in the body—the ill forces so to say—which cause the fever. The state of the urine is the result of the loss of valuable salts, tissues, etc., from the body, and largely explains the great weakness of the patient, his light-headedness, rambling, nightmares and so on; it also explains the long convalescence and bad after-effects in the case of patients who have been treated in the orthodox suppressive manner. The rational method of avoiding all this is urine-therapy so that the lost tissue may be replaced. I have proved it again and again to be successfully accomplished in diphtheria, chickenpox, scarlet fever, influenza, rheumatic fever, and other acute disorders where the temperature is high; and there have been none of those baneful and chronic after-effects which so often accrue after wrongly treated scarlet-fever or rheumatic fever; all of which are due to suppressive measures.

CHAPTER XI.

A Case of Orchitis

Orchitis is a most agonising complaint in which the testicles swell, and sometimes become ulcerated. It may be caused by injury, by gonorrhoea, or it may occur during an attack of mumps. In its most severe form, however, it is a comparatively rare disorder in this country (England). The doctor who was called in took a very serious view of this case, and gave the victim only a few days to live. When, after a journey away from home, I first saw the victim—aged 19—his bowels had not functioned for a week, and his kidneys for 72 hours. One side of his body was swollen as though someone had placed half a football under the flesh. His testicles were as large as tennis balls, and the glans penis was 14 inches in length, as solid as a lead pencil and twisted round like a corkscrew; moreover it had turned black. The victim's groans and writhings in agony were heartrending. Although for three days he had eaten nothing and had merely drunk pints of plain water, the swellings and distortions had only increased. As he had passed no urine of his own to drink, I was obliged to give him a pint of mine to take.

Two hours after the first draught, the glans penis showed signs of becoming so far normal that he was able to pass some urine in small drops—about two egg-cups full in all. It was thick, muddy and as concentrated as gruel mixed with blood, very dark and exceedingly malodourous. Nevertheless he drank it without a grimace or a murmur. Four hours later he passed nearly a pint of the same evil-looking and evil-smelling water: which he also drank without a grimace. He informed me that he could not taste it owing to the state of his palate due to the acids which rose from his stomach. This, by the way, is liable to occur in the course of a fast.

Two hours later the patient had a very copious and offensive stool, the equal of which I have not seen in all the 27 years' experience I have had in treating diseases. During the evacuation some urine was passed which the patient subsequently drank. Having carried him back to bed, we found that he could now lie comfortably stretched out, whereas, previously his knees had been drawn up to his abdomen, like people suffering from peritonitis or appendicitis. He was now nearly free from pain, precisely eight hours after he had taken the first draught of urine. I now laid cloths soaked in old urine on his abdomen, chest and head, and bound up his feet and hands in a similar manner. He passed more and more water, and drank every drop. His bowels responded to the treatment and worked freely and painlessly, the evacuations being not unlike discoloured water.

On the 4th day he passed 22 pints of urine in 24 hours: all of which he drank immediately.

And now came a set-back. On the fifth day I was called to Manchester on business, and in my absence a friendly doctor induced him to take a tablespoon of ground wheat in water. The result was disastrous. All flow of urine ceased, and in 16 hours all the previous symptoms had returned, though in a slightly less aggravated form. There was nothing for it but to begin the whole treatment over again.

The patient finally broke his fast on the 17th day with the juice of one orange at noon, one whole orange at 2 p.m. and one whole orange at 4 p.m. At 8 p.m. a full glass of fresh milk. He slept soundly that night.

From the 18th to the 25th day his diet consisted of such foods as cold beef, steamed fish, potatoes in their

71

jackets, scrambled and poached eggs, pears and other fresh fruits, salads, tomatoes—and nothing else.

On the 26th day the patient was back at his work, completely cured. That was many years ago. He is now a man of forty, lives on a well-balanced diet, drinks his own " water of life, " and enjoys perfect health.

I may mention that the late Dr. Rabagliati was so impressed with this case that he wrote a detailed account of it which was sent to four medical journals in England and U.S.A. Not one of them would publish it. Allusions to cures effected by laymen are not welcomed by medical journals. Medical publications have policies just like daily papers The fact that a thing may be true or useful to the helping of their fellows seem to play a secondary part with editors of medical papers of the orthodox variety. This is unfortunate, as it is of course obstructive to progress and medical enlightenment, a matter which was recognised by the Health Practitioners' Association. Indeed, in the *Health Practitioners' Journal,* we find articles by homoeopaths, naturopaths, herbalists, osteopaths, yoga practitioners, biologists, biochemists, etc., etc.—the laudable belief being that there are many roads to health and many means of treating disease.

CHAPTER XII.

VENEREAL DISEASES

Drs. Bosanquet and Eyre in their book entitled *Serums, Vaccines and Toxins* were constrained to admit: " It cannot be denied that in a certain number of instances the injection of diphtherial anti-toxin has been followed by death directly attributable to the action of the serum. " One of these tragedies, the earliest and perhaps the saddest befell Dr. Langenhans of Berlin. Because one of his servants developed diphtheria, as a precautionary measure, he inoculated his perfectly healthy child of one year nine months old. In a few moments the unfortunate child was dead. The irony of it is that there was not the slightest evidence to prove that the child would ever have contracted the disease, seeing that diphtheria germs may be found in a number of quite healthy throats, and in such an environment are as harmless as are many another supposed-to-be deadly germs. But, alas it is not merely injections for diphtheria that have proved fatal, for hundreds of deaths, many of them instantaneous, resulted from the use of *salvarsan,* otherwise called " 606 " in the treatment of syphilis. Nevertheless, just as immunisation against diphtheria is boosted, *salvarsan* was boosted as the cure *par excellence* for venereal disease.

Of syphilis we read: " Whether he has been treated or not, the patient is always liable to develop nerve symptoms. These are the most serious of all the complications of syphilis and the commonest are general paralysis and locomotor ataxia. They usually show themselves about ten years after infection. In general paralysis there is progressive dementia, usually with some form of exaltation. The speech is hesitating, slurred and tremulous. The face muscles and tongue show paresis with tremors .... Later the muscular powers become gradually weakened until there is more or less general paralysis .... " (Dr. E. H. Ruddock, M.D.) This is a most unpleasant and saddening picture. Yet I suggest that the horrible after-effects of venereal disease are the result of suppressive treatment. What after all is syphilis? It is simply the result of a poison which is absorbed into the body, and hence the rational treatment is to get that poison *out* of the body.

As the Medical Profession reserves the right to treat venereal diseases, and has its clinics for that purpose, I as a layman, or a naturopath as I am sometimes called, am prohibited from treating it. All the same there are men, who having heard of urine-therapy through the late Mr. Baxter's pamphlets (mentioned in Chapter II) and through other channels, have set about treating themselves.

I will here give the case of a man who contracted venereal disease in France during the last war (1918). He had, by the way, suffered for some time from psoriasis, which he had suppressed with herbal ointments. This man, then still young, knew something about Nature-cure methods and had endeavoured to treat his venereal disease by subsisting for a time entirely on cold water in the hope of " starving it out. " At the end of an 11 days' fast, however, his symptoms, far from being better, were decidedly worse. It was then that he came across one of the Baxter booklets. The upshot was that he decided to continue the fast, but be it noted, with the addition of the internal and external use of his own urine. The results were gratifying in the extreme; at the end of ten days every sign of the venereal disease had vanished, and the psoriasis had greatly improved. Nevertheless, he decided to continue the urine-fast until all traces of the

74

skin complaint had disappeared. This eventuated in one more week, and he found himself free of all his troubles. And not only that, but he also found that his sight, hearing, senses of taste and smell had become more acute than they had been for years.

Most people are now familiar with the orthodox methods of dealing with venereal disease. Sufferers are invited to attend clinics where they are treated with injections. The treatment may last over a period of either weeks or months. But although members of the poorer classes may attend these clinics, notabilities, particularly in the smaller towns, prefer to be treated by their own doctors, as they feel a certain embarrassment at showing themselves in a place where they may be recognised. In any event, the grave question one asks oneself is: What will be the after-effects of these injections? It is one thing to treat the disease, but that is not the same as permanently curing the *patient.* Wrote Dr. W. H White, M.D., of Orthodoxy: " Medicine ignores the individual ' wholeness ' and treats the disease as a *separate entity."* Thus there are remedies tabulated for practically any ailment from rheumatism to syphilis: but as the homoeopath points out, what the allopath calls rheumatism may come from twenty different causes (were he to say from twenty different secondary *causes,* this would more approximate to the truth) hence the name of the disease is of really no importance. Regarded from my particular · point of view, I would even add "nor how it has been contracted" for the method of cure, as I have shown, is the same.

To revert to the case of venereal disease I have cited. If the young man in question had employed urine-therapy from the first instead of trying to treat it with what are termed nature-cure methods, I am convinced that it would have been cured far sooner. From what I have been able to gather from others who have tried urine-therapy on

75

their own, I have good reason to believe that where venereal disease has been taken in its initial stage, or during the first week, cures have been effected anywhere from between 48 to 96 hours; that is provided it has not been complicated by the usual treatment. But of course as it is illegal for me to treat this age-old affliction I am in no position to furnish case-histories. Still, to exclude from these pages mention of such diseases as the Medical Profession reserve the right to treat by their own methods would be to leave my task only half fulfilled. Considering that " a proportion of all the blind, the deaf, the mentally deficient and the crippled owe their disabilities to venereal diseases " (see *Britain's Health*) it becomes the duty of any one, be he doctor or layman, who has found a means of curing it, to make his discovery known so that doctors can make use of it if they wish. What we have to remember is that measures employed for treating venereal diseases, as most others also, have their day, are found perhaps to be unsatisfactory, and then are superceded by other methods. Although it is doubtful whether the clinics will be prepared to try urine-therapy, there may be some private doctors who may be willing to give it a trial. Time alone can show. I may add, by the way, that although doctors do not realise the full value of urine, there are those who have pointed out that if only men would micturate immediately after coitus, the risk of contracting venereal disease would be minimised. The late Mr. Baxter, J.P., was right when he published the fact that among other things urine possessed strong antiseptic properties.

CHAPTER XIII.

The Cure of Wounds which would not Heal: The Treatment of Burns.

I was destined to prove the value of urine-therapy in the treatment of wounds, when some years ago through an accident I suffered a grave laceration and injury to my toes, ankle and foot. The toe-nails were torn off and the toes forced back into the fleshy part of the foot. Naturally the shock and pain were very severe. All the same I rejected the help of a medical friend, as I was resolved once again to prove the effects of urine-treatment on wounds.

After having the damaged portions of my foot put into place by some Physical Culture practitioners who had witnessed the accident, I fasted four days for the shock (an approved method) and applied cloths saturated in old urine to the affected parts. These bandages were kept moist by repeated soakings; but were not unwound until the fifth day. When finally removed, the results were astonishing; all trace of the injury had disappeared, and the foot was healthy and supple as it had been in early youth. Incidentally a corn which had troubled me was dissolved by the treatment.

I have frequently observed similar effects even on wounds which had refused to heal, whether under the treatment of common medical, herbal or other remedies, and even where amputation had been seriously discussed as the only remaining course to pursue.

From among the large number of cases I have treated. I will now give the history of a particularly bad one, which came under my care in 1918. In that year, I was introduced to a man in the early forties who at the time was attending the local Infirmary as an out-patient every week for a bullet-wound in the fore-arm. Although the patient had received the wound a year previously, it had shown no signs of healing, was about 10 inches in length, about three-eights of an inch in width, and at times ulcerous and suppurating. His medical advisers were afraid it might ultimately turn gangrenous, to avoid which, poisonous ointments and dressings were applied, with many changes in the ingredients and proportions in the mixings. Having got sick of orthodox methods, the patient had also resorted to Fletcherism and the Salisbury Treatment, from which admittedly he had derived some benefit; but even so that wound refused to heal. In spite of objections from his wife, he eventually became my patient.

My assistants first set about ripping off all the dressings. Then we washed the wounded arm three times a day with old urine, giving the rest of the body lengthy periods of massage with the bare hands and the same species of urine. The patient was fasted for three days on his own urine plus cold water, short spells of sun-bathing were advocated—and at the end of seven more days nothing remained of the fissure but a very slight scar as thin as a gold thread. In short, after a whole year's " interference treatment " the patient was cured by Nature in ten days!

Since the date of this cure I have observed scores of cases of " miraculous " healing by identically the same method; these include the healing of painful and disabling wounds, cuts, sores, ill-effects from rusty nails, fishbones, etc., also poisonous wounds and blood-poisoning generally. As a rule a long penance was not required. Cases taken early have responded to three or four days' treatment, whilst those which have been medically interfered with and almost rendered gangrenous have taken from ten to eighteen days.

With regard to burns, one reads that in a given year 7,900 Americans—almost half the number of which were children under five, died of burns. (Or did they die of the treatment or of both combined?) As to thousands of Americans who survived the effects of burns they were destined to suffer from unsightly scars, tight puckered skin, stiffened limbs or useless limbs and fingers.

For years the standby among remedies for burns was the application of wet tea-leaves. Then in 1925, Dr. Davidson of Detroit placed the old wives' remedy on a quasi scientific basis. Instead of the boiled tea-leaves, he applied the element derived therefrom which as we all know is called tannic acid. This poisonous substance literally tans the tissues, and a thick, hard crust then forms over the exposed nerve ends. But although it relieves the pains it checks the activity and flow of the body fluids to the parts, the while it acts as a covering under which it is hoped that new skin may form. Unfortunately, however, the tannic acid not only "tans" the burned tissues, but also the surrounding healthy tissues, with the result that it destroys cells which ought to be providing new cells for the knitting together of the skin elements—if I may thus express it for the benefit of the lay mind. The final outcome is a disfiguring scar, which is preventable by natural methods as opposed to "scientific" ones. Tannic acid is not even bacterial, for if foreign matter lurks on the burned surface, the function of the microscopic scavengers, which science calls germs, is impeded, and infection is more likely to persist under the supposedly protective crust. In the attempt to kill germs, we merely manacle the policeman!

The tannic acid treatment of burns was superceded by the picric acid treatment, and also the acriflavine treatment. Then the surgeons tried *their* methods; they took skin from another part of the body—usually the buttocks —and grafted it onto the burnt portions. But unfortunately, it sometimes occurred that the wound left by the removal of the healthy tissue turned septic. As to the suffering for the patient which this method entails, it can be better imagined than described. Not that I wish to decry surgery where in the case of accidents and mutilation from war it is necessary. But I am constrained to say that surgery has greatly been abused, and continues to be abused, and thousands of unneeded operations are performed on organs which could be treated by natural methods.

Nevertheless, some doctors have been broad-minded and enterprising enough to try urine-therapy, as witness the following extract from a letter to me in 1935 by Dr. Geo. S. Cotton of Temple, Texas, U.S.A.

" .... Since receiving your literature some months ago, I have put it (urine-therapy) to the test and the results have been astonishing. Urine in the treatment of wounds, etc., cannot be beaten. This healing power is brought about among other elements contained in urine, by ' Allontain ' ($C_4.H_6,O_3.N_4$).

" As I put urine to further use in the treatment and eradication of disease, I shall send you full information. It appears to me you are furthering a great truth which should be broadcast to suffering humanity .... "

CHAPTER XIV.

SOME MISCELLANEOUS CASES.

Enuresis nocturna (bed-wetting). Sometimes this is merely a bad habit, but more generally it is a morbid symptom in nervous and anaemic children. Weakness is the principal cause, although it may also be due to worms. Children are supposed to grow out of this distressing condition, but this is not always the case.

Boy, aged 9, had suffered from enuresis all his young life, and had been treated by physicians both of the orthodox and unorthodox schools. Was very thin, and very unhappy about his affliction. Fasted on urine for 11 days. Result, complete cure.

Menstruational Trouble. The patient had suffered for over two years from too prolonged and too frequent menstruation, for which she had first tried allopathy without effect, and then herbalism, from which she only obtained partial relief. The complaint was not only weakening her physically but was also affecting her mental equilibrium. During one of her long periods which had already lasted a fortnight, she decided to try urine-therapy. Although at first the urine was heavily over-charged with menstrual blood, she was nevertheless heroic enough to take it. During her fast she also sipped from two or three pints daily of plain cold water. In three days the urine became normal. She continued the fast for exactly 28 days, during which she was rubbed with a healthy person's urine for some hours each day. The case was a complete cure not only of the menstrual trouble but also of long standing nasal catarrh, and an increasing tendency to deafness.

81

Nephritis with other distressing symptoms. Young woman. Had been in the care of two doctors for some weeks, and had also seen a specialist, who told her mother that the case was a hopeless one, and that in all probability this particular victim would not live to see the approaching Christmas. The young woman was then brought to me. To encourage her and induce her to take the offensive looking urine she passed, I even went so far as to drink a little of it myself. After a fast of 30 days on urine and cold water only, and daily rubbings with healthy urine, the patient was cured of her grievous complaint. Nor did any other malady develop subsequently. When I first saw her she had weighed 106 lbs.; four months later on a regime of two well-balanced meals a day, and the continued use internally and externally of her own urine, she weighed 136 lbs. nude, which is the normal weight for a woman of her height and build.

Mucus Colitis. Boy of 6, began to discharge mucus frequently, though otherwise there were no apparent symptoms of ill-health. The doctor, when sent for, said the trouble was prevalent, and prescribed castor oil. But the boy's father, who knew me and my methods, thinking a castor oil purge too violent, sent for me as soon as the doctor had gone. I put the boy on a urine fast, and in 48 hours all the trouble had disappeared. Nevertheless, as it is foolish to start eating as soon as symptoms vanish, the boy fasted four days in all.

Two days later, the boy's mother developed the same colitis symptoms, likewise did her sister. I fasted them both for eight days according to my method, though the actual symptoms vanished in five days or sooner. It is worthy of note that all three patients were strict vegetarians, and that the boy had never tasted flesh in his young life. I advised them to include some flesh food in their dietary.

Eye Injury. In 1920 a lady came to me with a splinter of chip-wood in one eye. The splinter had pierced the iris and was sticking out an inch or more. I removed the splinter, fasted the patient on urine and water for a few weeks, at the end of which time the trouble was completely cured and the patient had perfect sight.

Psoriasis. Gentleman, aged 60. Fasted on urine and water for one week in June, 1920, and again for one week in September of the same year. During and between the fasts, had rubbings of his own urine in spells of an hour three times a day. Complete cure. He continued the intake of urine as a daily habit, and ten years later, though three score years and ten, only looked about 56. I regard psoriasis and eczema as amongst the easiest diseases to cure by means of urine-therapy; that is provided they are taken in time. Nor is lupus, a more serious skin disease and said to be caused by the tubercle bacillus, by any means incurable, though the treatment takes longer.

Rheumatic fever followed by influenza. Female patient, 16 stone, though not a big eater, having lost two stone before I visited her. Heavily constipated, suffering from insomnia and worry. Bedfast with swollen hips, feet, ankles and abdomen. Fasted a week on urine and plain water, was well rubbed every day according to my usual method. Complete cure in a month, and back at her occupation.

Pyorrhoea. Patient was in the habit of visiting his dentist every six months. Dentist informed him that he was suffering from pyorrhoea. Having heard of urine-therapy, without telling his dentist, he took half a pint of his urine every morning and also urine as a mouth-wash. In nine weeks his trouble had completely disappeared, much to the surprise of his dentist, who wished to know what had caused such a marked improvement in his general health as to cure pyorrhoea. This cure was effected even without a fast. *(Case reported by a friend).*

The notion that pyorrhoea is a local disease for which one must have all the teeth extracted is a fallacy. There is no such thing as a local disease; there are only localised symptoms. Cleanse the body of its impurities by a fast on urine and plain water, and pyorrhoea vanishes automatically. I have observed this in numerous cases— in fact, in all cases I have ever treated. As for myself, I never require to visit a dentist; a well-balanced diet and urine-therapy have preserved my teeth.

Obesity. Married lady, aged 30, weighed 12 stone 6 lbs. Had no children. Lived on the usual ill-balanced diet, but was not a glutton, masticated her food, and drank only water, after or between meals. Previously she had tried various diets without effect, and had tried fasting on plain water only, but with the result that as soon as she resumed eating she put on weight even more rapidly than prior to the fast. Finally, she consulted me. I advised a urine plus plain water fast with daily rubbings, and at the end of 14 days her weight dropped to 10 stone. I then revised her diet, put her on to a well-balanced regime, and suggested two meals a day only. By dint of living in this way and taking her own urine daily, her weight has remained about 10 stone, and although she is now past 50, she looks about 33.

With many people obesity does not arise from over-indulgence at the table, but from badly functioning glands caused by toxins and a deficiency of the required elements which should be derived from non-processed foods. The fast cleanses the blood tissues, and the intake of urine brings back normality to the disordered glands. I have conclusively proved this by the large number of cases of obesity I have treated, or where obesity has been present among other symptoms.

Prostate Troubles. Enlargement of the prostate is a term referring to an affliction often to be met with in elderly men. " The most prominent symptom is an irritability of the bladder and a r~·~~essive incapacity to empty it. The prostate gland undergoes a considerable increase in size, and by pressing on the neck of the bladder forms an obstruction to the outflow of urine from that organ ... " (See E. H. Ruddock, M.D. *Vade Mecum.*)

Case of prostate trouble in its incipient stage. Old gentleman began to have difficulty in voiding his urine. Was advised by a friend to try taking half a pint of his own water every morning on rising; this to be followed at the usual time by a *light* breakfast instead of the customary full meal. Result: in one month after starting the treatment he was rid of his trouble.

Bronchial Asthma. Miss C. Doctor had diagnosed the case as bronchial catarrh; the victim said to be in the early stages of T.B. General health very poor. Breathing difficult. Victim had to resort to palliatives to obtain ease and short periods of much needed sleep. Felt very weak and debilitated. Heard of urine-therapy. Fasted for a fortnight on urine, but without the rubbings. In three days the improvement was so marked that she was able to breathe freely and sleep each night for several hours on end. Broke fast, took two meals a day only, and continued the intake of urine. But the fast had not been sufficiently long to eradicate the trouble and her symptoms returned. She then wrote to me for advice. I told her that she had not broken the fast correctly, advised further fasts *to be attended with the rubbings,* and gave her a diet to be followed between the fasts. The final result was a complete cure, and the patient has remained in excellent health. She continues to take her own urine daily, and from time to time resorts to short fasts, with the result that she feels better than she has ever done.

Case of gangrene and after-effects of drug-treatment for thyroid trouble.

(Reported by the Naturopath, Mr. O. Warnock-Fielden.) Lady aged 40. Long history of drug treatment since she was 15. In early life she had had injections during a number of years for over active thyroid, and also for colds. More recently she had had an operation with a view to improving the circulation, seeing that when the weather was cold, and even at other times, her hands would go blue. No improvement was noticed after the operation. Before I was called in, the local doctor had retired from the case, pronouncing it to be hopeless. I found her hands a mass of pus, moist gangrene, and almost skinless. The necessity for amputation of both hands had been mooted and feared. After making a start with less severe measures such as hot fomentations, cold compresses, urine-packs, urine drinking in small quantities, and an antiseptic ointment to relieve the intense " drawing " pains, I finally advocated a complete fast on urine and plain water only, at the same time continuing the packs. The fast lasted three weeks, but even after a fortnight, the patient could use her hands and could knit. Granted that the urine-drinking and the urine-dressings were of much value to the treatment, I none the less consider that the three weeks' fast was the decisive factor in this case, since it enabled the drug-laden system to be drained of its impurities.

Rash on the arms. Mrs. C. suffered for over three years from an irritating eruption on her arms. Had tried various ointments and lotions without any relief. Was finally induced to try the effect of urine, which she dabbed on every night. The rash disappeared completely within a few weeks. In this case no fasting was resorted to or any other measures.

Large wart on face. Mrs. C. reports that she employed the same treatment for an unsightly excrescence on her face, which in a short time shrivelled up and then fell away, leaving no scar. (All three of these cases were supplied by Mr. Warnock-Fielden.)

Lump on arm. A correspondent reports the case of a lady who developed a nasty blue looking lump about $\frac{1}{2}$ inch high, which she feared might become malignant. She was advised by an acquaintance to treat it with urine-compresses, and in less than three weeks it fell off, leaving the skin healthy and clean.

A mysterious case. Male patient about 58. Had been in the hospital for several weeks for observation and treatment, but at the end of the term was said to be incurable, and was sent home to die, but enjoined to keep in touch with his local doctor. He was given a particular drug to take with him which was calculated to dissolve any food he ate. When, at the request of a gentleman I was treating, I first saw the patient, I reckoned he was dying sure enough, but not from the disease so much as from the powerful drug (poison) he was being given. I noticed that his eye-balls were much distended, that he was thin, but not to the extent of emaciation. He told me he had been a careful eater, a hard outdoor worker, had kept regular hours, had never been subject to colds, had never been bilious or consti-pated and had never had diarrhoea. His only vice had been the use of snuff, but he had discontinued the habit a year previously. I only stayed with him a few minutes at my first visit, told him to fast and to drink nothing but cold water and every drop of urine that he passed both day and night. I also told him (and his wife) not to be surprised at any symptoms which might occur in the process of elimination. His stools and ejecta were to be kept for my inspection. Three days later I called again, to be shown two large buckets full of the foul matter he had vomited—the vomiting having started 24 hours after he had taken his first draught of urine. There had also been great looseness of the bowels, and much catarrhal discharge from the nose. In fact he had been obliged to use a dozen handkerchiefs, which were not only soiled with ropy mucus but also with SNUFF! The fast was continued, and in a week all discharge ceased. The penance was broken in 10 days—and the patient was cured. At the time of writing he is over 70. This case is interesting as it serves to show that with urine-therapy it is quite unnecessary to know the name of the disease in order to treat it. It is further interesting as showing that a foreign substance—snuff in this case—may be lodged in the tissues for months after the taking of it has been discontinued, only to be eliminated during a body-cleansing fast. Which reminds me that the eminent German naturopath, Louis Kuhne, relates of a case where during the eliminative treatment the sweat of the patient had smelt of drugs the allopaths had previously used to cure—or rather—*suppress* the disease. (See his *New Science of Healing*.)

Jaundice. It must be remembered that jaundice is merely a symptom of some chronic or acute affection of the liver and is not a disease in itself. My first and most difficult case where a jaundiced condition obtained was in 1919, at the beginning of my career as a urine-therapist. This case took 10 days to clear up on a urine-fast plus tap-water.

I have not had a number of jaundice cases; but with those I have treated it has been remarkable to watch the discolouration of the skin gradually disappear during the first two or three days of the fast, and then as the penance has continued, give place to a colour as fresh and healthy as the complexion of a diarymaid! Ten days or less have usually sufficed to clear up a jaundiced condition, that is provided it has not been due to cancer of the liver. This dread disease I regard as practically hopeless by whatever means it is treated. Even biochemic practitioners, who have claimed to cure some cases of cancer, maintain that if the liver is involved, nothing can be done. Nevertheless I once supervised a urine-fast in the case of a man who had been such a heavy drinker that over a period of years he had drunk a whole bottle of spirits per diem. This man decided to try a urine-fast while his doctor was away on holiday. He drank all the urine he voided, but on the tenth day it remained as bloody and as full of red sandy deposit as it was at the beginning of the penance. On the day in question the doctor returned from his holiday, and an incision was made in the scrotum. The following day the patient passed away in a state of unconsciousness. Whether his liver which was "dead" could ever have been made to function again if the fast had continued and there had been no surgical interference is very problematical; but I confess I was much distressed that at any rate I was not given the chance to *try* and save the unfortunate man's life, especially as during the fast he had lost very little flesh except in the face, and so there seemed some prospect of his ultimate recovery. And, after all, where there is life there is hope!

Case of paralysis, premature old age, loss of memory, etc. Male patient, aged 60. Medical verdict, "a few weeks to live." Had had two paralytic seizures, the first occurring after an attempt to get rid of influenza by means of fresh fruit and fruit juices. After the second seizure he had no memory, and appeared to be in his dotage, though only 60. He underwent a urine-fast.

89

with rubbings, for 59 days, broke the spell for a fortnight, living on the one meal a day plan, then fasted further for another 35 days. Memory and his speech returned in 20 days during the first fast, and the cure was completed during the second, the prime cause of the trouble having been an arthritic condition.

Loss of hair. This same man who had lost his hair, not only regained it during the second fast—his head was rubbed daily—but instead of being grey it assumed its original colour .... Many of my correspondents, I may add, report renewal of hair as the result of rubbing the head with *old* urine as a daily habit.

Reports from correspondents on influenza, pneumonia, pleurisy and appendicitis.

These reports show that as a general rule from three to eight days' urine-fast suffices to cure influenza, pneumonia and pleurisy. The same can be said of appendicitis. In some cases of the latter, one small meal a day has been allowed, though all the urine passed must be taken. In severe acute cases with fever, a complete urine-fast is essential.

And here I would emphasise the fact that to press food on a sick man or woman on the principle that strength *must* be kept up, is the height of medical folly. To an invalid whose instincts and organs rebel against taking nourishment, food acts like a poison.

Cataract. Before it became illegal for laymen to mention the fact that cataract may yield to treatment without operation, I found that in many cases, 10 days' urine-fast was sufficient to dissolve the film that forms over the eye. The longest required was a 28 days' fast. Whether it is against the now existing law for any layman to say that he *has* cured cataract *before* the law was passed, is a subtle point on which I am not qualified to pronounce. But in case the disclosure should be illegal, we must assume that the cases cured had been falsely diagnosed, since the law implies that no one save a qualified oculist can cure genuine cases, namely with a knife. Nevertheless, it is only veracious to say that cataract is by no means always an isolated condition. What we need to remember is that the eye is a part of the body, and therefore in treating the body as a whole for other symptoms, the local condition is apt to cure itself without any direct attention.

Glaucoma. This, according to orthodox Medicine and even to naturopathy, is a very serious condition. Oculists perform an operation, but in many cases the patient sooner or later merely goes blind. In any event, mutilation can never be termed a cure. Patients who have not been tampered with, I have known to respond well on a urine-fast of about a month's duration. As against that, cases which have been surgically interfered with must as a general rule be considered practically hopeless.

Rheumatism. In this country (England) the weather is often blamed for rheumatic conditions by persons with insufficiently alkaline blood. But were the blood and body free from acidity and foreign matter, the weather or changes of weather would have no effect.

With regard to the cure for rheumatism (of which some doctors say there are 26 different kinds) I have found that patients always respond well to a urine-fast of from 10 to 12 days, or even less in simple cases. The fast must be attended with the urine-rubbings and urine-packs. After the cure, revision of diet to a well balanced regime is essential to avoid recurrence. Many cases have even responded to the one meal a day plan (the food must be carefully chosen, alcohol and condiments avoided) plus the taking of autogenous urine, the urine-rubbings, and urine-packs. Such cases, if of not too long-standing and severe, have usually cleared up within a few weeks.

Arthritis. This painful and distressing condition is about as far removed from rheumatism as a severe attack of influenza from a slight cold, and is one of the very worst conditions to tackle; notably because the foreign deposits are largely lodged in the *bones.* Even to cure *an incipient case* I have found that it takes anywhere from 12 to 40 days on a very carefully selected diet, the taking of every drop of urine passed, and long daily rubbings with urine. (These were cases where the patients had objected to or had not found it feasible to fast.) Nevertheless, I regard such treatment as only half measures, and maintain that a complete urine-fast of even 10 days does far more to help the victims than months of mere dieting and the taking of urine. But I must emphasise that where the trouble has become deep-seated, and the victim is practically crippled, there is little prospect of obtaining a cure.

I will now add a few cases kindly supplied by the naturopath Mr. Oliver Warnock-Fielden:

"Bronchial Asthma. Mr. D.E., age 37. Discharged from the Navy for Bronchial Asthma, from which he had suffered since the age of 14. The sea life seemed to make the trouble worse. Disturbed each night at least four times in order to use a medical spray, also he dare not go to the theatre without it so that he could use it between the acts. Within three months, during which he drank urine up to three or four pints a day, and two short fasts of 36 to 40 hours each on urine alone, he became so much relieved that he never thinks of taking his spray to the theatre, nor does he wake up at night to use it. All fear of his trouble has left him and his general health is vastly improved.

Another case of the same trouble improved in a four

92

days' fast on urine, when a three weeks' fast at a well-known Nature Cure Home had utterly failed. After every drink of urine a wad of mucus was discharged. The last day of the fast produced such a clot of mucus that the patient went out and tested his breathing by walking up a hill. Experiencing no difficulty he immediately returned to work."

"Diseased Kidney. Mr. G.D. In May, 1944, he was in hospital for the removal of his right kidney. He had suffered great pain, the urine was the colour of blood, and the X-ray had shown a large stone lodged in the pelvis of the kidney. The surgeon's opinion was that the kidney was diseased and not to remove it would be a danger to life. However, Mr. D. refused the operation and came to me. He took to urine drinking quite naturally, drank all he passed, fasted repeatedly for several days at a time, and within a few weeks the condition was improved to the extent that there was no pain and the urine was of normal colour. In three months Mr. D. returned to the hospital and was told that there was nothing wrong with his kidney.

As a result of this successful treatment, Mr. D. brought me a patient who had been in hospital waiting to undergo the same operation. He also was cured by the same method.

In cases such as these one must accept the verdict of the examining surgeons and the radiologist who in both instances were pressing for an operation as the only means of relief, or even of saving life. When later on they maintain that there is nothing at all wrong, and the X-ray gives a clear proof of a healthy kidney, one is forced to assume that the fasting and urine drinking has effected the cure."

To conclude this chapter I may append one or two suggestions made by my friend Mr. O. Warnock-Fielden as to how urine cures, although I may not altogether share his views. He writes:

" There may be some healing force in the return of the unexpected hormones particularly the sex hormones, which find their way into the urine. There are cases known in which urine is taken internally for the sake of these substances alone. There may also be a case made out for the return of the tissue substance which is in solution in the urine. Organic tissue may be leeched from the vital organs by means of the poisonous substances lodged there from the food and drink taken into the body, and also from the drugs and injections of medical science. It is claimed by some that these substances may be returned and used again in re-building healthy organs. This is difficult to prove, but there are many cases on record in which diseased organs have been renewed by means of drinking large quantities of urine. More than this it is impossible to say."

" The explanation which appeals to me more than any other is that cures are obtained by means of the homoeopathic principle. There is no doubt that although it is claimed that toxic matter in quantity is not thrown out of the body in the urine (otherwise we would not become ill because it remains in) there must certainly be found in all urine a homoeopathic, or infinitesimal dose of the particular toxic complex of the individual concerned. That must surely be beyond all argument. If this infinitesimal dose is returned to the body, an antibody, according to homoeopathic principles, will be produced, and will therefore tend towards a cure of the condition. "

" In the natural habits of animals we observe the fact that they continually lick themselves. In this way they undoubtedly take into their systems homoeopathic doses of their toxic condition. After every meal, even, this dose would tend to correct any harm likely to occur from eating food which would not agree with them, perhaps even poison them. May not this habit be Nature's immunisation scheme *par excellence?* Medical science has formulated a system of dangerous inoculations to do exactly the same thing as the dog does when it licks itself. Nature gives instinct to the dog for its salvation, and brains to man for his ultimate destruction! We may be too clever. If anyone doubts the animal's instinct to drink its own urine, let him try the experiment of handing a cup to a monkey. The monkey has only one use for it. The goat is considered to be the most healthy of all animals, so much so that its milk is much sought after for T.B. cases. May not this be explained by the fact that the goat can, and very often does, drink its urine straight from its body? "

" When man first appeared upon the earth, some provision must have been made for his security against extinction. Food, clothing, shelter were all stored within the earth, man having only to work for them to satisfy all his material needs. Would the vital importance of his freedom from disease be neglected? If what is stated in these pages is correct, the means whereby health may be attained is always close at hand, easy to carry out, marvellous in its simplicity and free to everyone. The late Dr. Chas. H. Duncan, one of the most enlightened doctors of America, states in his book *Autotherapy:*

' There are in the pathogenic exudates toxic substances to which the patient must develop resistance in order that a cure may be instituted. In other words, in Autotherapy the patient has the right toxic substances within his body, and it remains for the physician to find them and determine the proper dose and the interval between doses so that the local tissues may develop resistance to them. '

There is therefore, much in some branches of medical

research which agrees with the courageous contribution of John Armstrong which is testified to in the cases mentioned in this book. "

CHAPTER XV.

THE COMMON COLD

It is not extravagant to say that the simple malady we call an ordinary common cold has baffled the Profession for centuries. A doctor once said to the writer: " If there is one thing I dislike being asked to cure, it is a common or garden cold in the head!" The late Dr. Haig, who first drew attention to uric acid, and better still to the folly of living on an unbalanced diet (though on certain points one might differ from him) told people they should be thankful when they contracted a streaming cold, as it acted as a species of house-cleaning, and therefore should never be suppressed. But unfortunately for mankind at large, very often the first thing most persons do immediately they " begin to feel a cold coming on" is to buy something to stop it, and " nip it in the bud. " This is not curing it, it is merely suppressing it and frustrating Nature. The suppression of a simple cold often leads to worse afflictions, such as pneumonia, etc.

The cause of colds is as simple as colds themselves are common; it lies in an unbalanced diet, and as the majority of people live on unbalanced diets, the majority of people are thus in varying degrees susceptible to colds. Excess of starch in a diet combined with a deficiency of foods containing the essential mineral salts is productive of catarrh. The exudations in catarrhal conditions should in themselves be quite sufficient to indicate to us the real cause of catarrh—*their nature is starchy*. Moreover, just as the cause of a cold must be obvious, so must be its cure, as I have found through years of observation and experience.

The procedure is to fast on cold water and self-urine only. No medicaments, whether in the form of lozenges or potions, must be taken. If this treatment is carried out, the cold will disappear, in the case of otherwise healthy individuals, in about 12 hours or less. Doubtless the reader will say: " but this is quite contrary to the old adage ' Feed a cold, and starve a fever '. " Yet was that the original adage? I have heard it said that such is merely a perversion of the original saying, which was: " If you feed a cold, you'll have to starve a fever. " Even a fast on cold water only will cure a cold in anything from 24 to 48 hours. But this is less effective than the cold water and self-urine treatment, which not only results in the rapid disappearance of the catarrhal condition, but the victim feels much better in every way than prior to the visitation. Moreover, which is very important, it prevents the development of influenza, pneumonia, etc., which when once developed may in some cases need at least a fast of 10 days, and much care and nursing.

And yet influenza, pneumonia, bronchitis and kindred ailments may be merely the more immediate results of suppressing Nature's attempts to get rid of an excess of starch and its evils. Indeed, it is my conviction that suppressed colds are the most fruitful and common basis of a long list of major diseases. Coryza, as it is technically called, i.e., the inflammation of the mucus membrane of the nose, should be regarded as a blessing in disguise, for it is, so to say, the alarm-bell which announces that the interior needs a cleansing process. And I would here stress at the risk of repetition that nothing performs this office so quickly, easily and actively as the intake of every drop of one's own urine *while fasting,* even if the passing and intake of that urine is up to 20 pints in the 24 hours of a fast.

As to chronic nasal catarrh, those people who live on an unbalanced diet should be thankful for this "safety valve" which may prevent them from developing far more serious ailments. Those who attempt to suppress it by unnatural means may have to face serious consequences. Its cause is to be found in the habitual consumption of too much bread, especially white, of buns, scones, polished rice puddings, porridge, biscuits, especially made of white flour, and other starch foods. Where these aliments preponderate in a dietary it also involves a deficiency in those foods rich in the essential mineral salts. To say that sugars and starch give energy is one of those pernicious half-truths which are nearly as misleading as a 100 per cent error. An *excess* of starch cannot give energy, because it merely clogs the system and inhibits its normal functioning. The proof is that people who live mostly on the aliments I have enumerated, have constantly to resort to alcoholic beverages or cups of tea to "buck themselves up."

As I always like to substantiate my contentions with scientific reasons for the benefit of those who like the i-s dotted in this manner, I may add that apart from an excess of starch being the cause of catarrh, there is in the tissues a deficiency of chloride of potash, phosphate of lime and sulphate of lime, and if the throat is infected, of phosphate of iron. (See *Biochemic Pocket Book*, by E. F. W. Powell, D.Sc.) In recent times researchers have occupied themselves with the analysis of various foods in order to ascertain their mineral-salts content. As a result of this, we find that some foods are richer in one or other salt than other foods. Thus the aliments have been tabulated under such headings as Carbon Foods, Calcium Foods, Chlorine Foods, Flourine Foods,

Sodium Foods, Potassium Foods, Phophorus Foods, Sulphur Foods, etc., etc. As all these salts have now been found to be essential to the proper functioning of the body, such research only serves again to show how necessary it is to live on a varied and well-balanced diet. It is significant that until recently, the Medical Profession ignored Potassium (potash) as a salt of any importance to the human body. And yet it has since been discovered by exponents of the Biochemic System that a deficiency of one or other forms of potash is a contributing cause in most diseases—especially in cancer and growths. Nevertheless, this was already discovered by Dr. Schuessler, of Oldenburg, Germany, in the latter half of last century. Yet it was only brought into greater prominence in 1912 by Dr. Forbes-Ross (already mentioned) who had probably never even heard of Dr. Schuessler or of his momentous but largely ignored discovery. In his General Sketch of *The Biochemic System of Medicine* G. W. Carey, M.D., significantly points out that a lack of any of the inorganic cell salts will set up certain symptoms which are merely Nature's method of indicating that one or more of the vital workers of the body are absent and must be supplied. " Each mineral salt has a special work to do. Each has an affinity for certain organic materials used in building up the human frame. Thus, Kali mur (chloride of potash) molecules work with fibrin. If a deficiency occurs in this salt, a portion of the fibrin not having inorganic salt to unite with becomes a disturbing element and may be thrown out of the vital circulation through the nasal passages or lungs ... producing conditions called catarrhs, colds, coughs, etc. "

Here, then, we have the biochemic explanation of colds and kindred ailments such as leucorrhoea (the whites) which when the discharge is milky white, indicates a deficiency of chloride of potash in the female organism.

(Carey.) I think I have now produced sufficient evidence to show that the common cold together with all catarrhal conditions, whether acute or chronic, is primarily the result of *wrong feeding*, on which I shall enlarge in a later chapter.

CHAPTER XVI.

Urine-Therapy on Animals

When certain people want to disparage a given treatment they ascribe its efficacy to Faith. For instance some opponents of homoeopathy have glibly dismissed it as a "faith-cure." Yet the homoeopath has an argument to hand which soon squashes that assumption; he contends that homoeopathy cures animals when in the nature of things they cannot know they are being treated. Cures of hundreds of animals are mentioned in homoeopathic literature. One is of a cat which had paralysis of its hind legs. After various treatments had been tried, its owner gave it *mag. phos* in a colossally high attenuation, and cured it completely in a very short time. The sceptic will say "coincidence." To which one can only retort: "How astonishing is the credulity of the sceptic!"

This allusion to homoeopathy on animals is so far relevant in that one or two "credulous sceptics" have even said that urine-therapy must be a "faith-cure." I can but smile and employ the same argument as have the homoeopaths. Let me substantiate my argument with a few facts.

It so happens that my grandfather was rather well known in the sixties and seventies of last century for his way with horses, dogs, etc., and it was from him I learned that urine and even cow-dung were his favourite remedies in successfully treating the ailments and injuries of animals. He thought nothing of fasting cows, horses and dogs up to a month on water and cow's urine, to administer which he used a horn; though when thirsty they would drink without this adjunct. Having learnt much from my grandfather, I treated animals myself. It was often a long and laborious job, and some adventures I could quote are not without their humorous side. I remember I once fasted a cow, which had tetanus, for 120 days, during which I rubbed it for eight hours a day with the urine (caught in buckets) of other cows. To drink I gave it its own urine (at first it was thick, yellow and concentrated as mustard) and the urine of healthy cows. It also drank plain cold water. My vaccine patient lost all its hair, went to skin and bone, but made a complete recovery, regaining its natural weight on grass-feeding in about two months.

I have also treated dogs by the urine-therapy fast. One method of inducing a dog to drink urine (though they will often drink a bitch's urine) is to fasten the animal to a tree and then syringe its head with a fine spray of the vital fluid. I used my own newly passed for the purpose. As the urine drips down over its face the dog will lap it up.

Case-history. Airedale terrier " Rough. " Treated him for a swelling in his abdomen which developed after he had been run over by the back wheel of a motorcar. He fasted 19 days on my urine and cold water when desired, and finally broke his fast on a little raw beef. When animals are ill, they have the sense to fast until hunger reasserts itself. During his fast I washed him all over with old, strong, greasy urine, and although he lost many of his old hairs during the process, he finished up with a beautiful coat.

Although the following experience with poultry does not strictly come under the heading of urine-therapy, since hens do not urinate and no urine was used, it is instructive none the less as showing what a fast will do even for birds. I had 60 hens at the time (October, 1916)

103

but not one of them had laid an egg for weeks, although they had been well fed and stimulated with condiments. As some of them were ill, many " authorities " had given me free or professional advice. Finally, I decided to put half of them on a fast, with nothing but plain water. The result was remarkable, for on the fourth day I found several eggs. Subsequently, I fasted the remaining half, with the same gratifying result—eggs in plenty. The fast in each case lasted a week. I then changed what had been the previous diet consisting of " anything and everything " to nothing but whole grain wheat—for which the hens had to work in ashes for every morsel—and *raw* greens, which I gave them twice a day. This, plus the grass they could peck from my orchards was all they got. The result was an average of 250 eggs a week from 60 hens for 18 weeks without a break, and at the negligible cost of ⅜d. per egg.

Treatment of a foal's leg for laceration. The foal in question had tried to force her way through a thick thorn hedge with disastrous results. She suffered a large slash in the flesh of one of her back legs at the knee-joint, and the gash resembled a great lip hanging down. I was advised to call in a vet. and have it stitched up, but I declined, knowing that such a measure would only leave unsightly marks and much reduce her value. I therefore bound up the wound with a soft clean woollen cloth (undyed) under a piece of three-ply flexible wood, and filled up the space between the flesh and the wood with cow-dung, finally drawing the poultice tight at the bottom with broad tape so as to keep the dung in place and let the foal have her run. Twice a day I called the animal so that I might pour a pint or more of urine into the top of the poultice in order to keep the properties of the dung active. This process I kept up for a fortnight. Then at length I undid the bandages—and lo and behold! the wound was perfectly healed, and without leaving a trace of a scar.

Truly there are lessons to be learnt from Nature. The first, second and third are—work with Nature and she will do the work!

CHAPTER XVII.

The Rationale of Rubbing and Urine Packs

A correspondent who asked a number of intelligent questions surprised me on that account by asking: " Is not the skin a one-way organ? " And yet what shred of evidence or deduction is there on which to base such an assumption? Take the simplest analogy. If one covers with a distended handkerchief the top of a cup containing a little milk, and then inverts the cup, the milk will ooze out through the handkerchief. Conversely, if one puts a little milk on the handkerchief distended over the cup, the milk will ooze through into the cup, and the more quickly if one rubs it through the material. That the skin is capable of absorbing not only fluids but air has been known for very many years. Why are cellular underclothes advocated? Because the skin requires to breathe. Hence the unwisdom of clogging the pores with suppressive unguents, or of " wrapping oneself up " in sheaths of warm underclothes, as did the Victorians. Should the skin be prevented from breathing entirely the victim dies. The story of the child which was painted completely with liquid gold in order to cut a figure in a pageant is well known—the child was dead in two hours. On the other hand the rubbing with milk of underweight and ill-thriving children was at one time a common practice, and often attended with good results. As we all know, friction produces heat, and heat opens up the pores of the skin because they likewise generate heat. That is why it is so important what the compresses contain. Compresses which merely draw out and put nothing back can prove seriously strength-sapping; a matter which has been brought to my notice in many cases. Thus the compress *par excellence* is a urine compress, and rubbing with urine is far superior to any other form of friction. For the latter purpose old urine alone, or old mixed with fresh, and warmed up (it must never be boiled) is the most efficacious. The most practical method is to store up urine in bottles, pour a very little into a flat-bottomed bowl, place the hands in the bowl so as to get just sufficient of the fluid on the palms, and then start the rubbing till the hands are dry. Pour a little more urine into the bowl, and repeat the process. By dint of taking only a little at a time on one's hands, none of the urine drops on to the floor.

As to compresses, from all that has already been written in this book when relating case-histories, how and when to apply them will have become obvious. However, it will do no harm to repeat myself. Cloths soaked in urine should be placed over the local site of the trouble, and kept moist by adding more urine when required. They should be applied wherever there are boils, burns, wounds, lumps, swellings, or other aberations. Naturally, the body will not be rubbed at the actual place where a compress is required. In no circumstances should suspicious lumps be rubbed or the tissues in the near vicinity.

I have already mentioned briefly that the most important parts to rub are the neck, face, head and feet. But that does not mean to say that the whole body should not be rubbed as well. Unless the malady requires a compress at one or other site, this is an essential part of urine-therapy in order to supply nourishment to the patient during a urine-fast. Apart from that, urine is the most wonderful skin-food that exists; as may be seen from the hands of those who do the rubbings.

It has been suggested by sceptics that a dry rub or a rub with plain cold water would be equally effective. But the answer is an emphatic negative. I have tried both. Even urine-fasts *without* the urine rubbings are attended with palpitations, just as are fasts on plain water only. I grant that the rubbing is both excellent exercise and acts as excellent massage, but without the urine it does not and cannot rebuild wasted tissues. Only in very bad cases where the patient is too weak and emaciated to stand it, have I dispensed with the rubbings, in which case the urine can be absorbed via the skin by means of the urine packs.

I will now give a case-history to show that continued poulticing with any other substance, however apparently harmless, can prove highly strength-sapping to the patient as well as quite unproductive of a cure.

Gentleman, well over 50. Had been an enthusiastic follower of what may be called a "caterpillar diet" It consisted of one meal a day, chiefly of wholemeal bread, salads, fresh fruits, fresh milk, nuts and honey. He had by this means hoped to reduce his "corporation" and to cure an arthiritic and dropsical condition and other troubles as well—chronic costiveness being one; for which he resorted to salts and high enemata. When he finally sent for me, he had been in the doctor's hands for some time, and was in such a state that he had to have two nurses. Although now taking two meals and four snacks a day, he was under 10 stone, very weak, bedfast, suffering from bed-sores, and spending half the day and most of the night coughing up phlegm and ropy mucus. But what I would draw special attention to here, was the state of his arm. About two years previously a running sore had manifested itself, to which poultices had been applied. In spite of this (or in my opinion largely because of it) he now had five discharging sores: the poulticing having been continued all that time (two years). I at once suggested that all this poulticing was responsible more than any other factor for his loss of strength, in that the constant "draining" of nourishment *via* his arm was starving both his limb and his torso. The upshot was—though the nurse protested—that the poulticing ceased, and the arm was simply bound in plain unmedicated rag, and not touched for a week. His meals were regulated to two a day, with no snacks, and only plain cool water to drink. All medicines (they had merely upset his digestion) were discarded. At the end of a week, the plain bandages were removed for inspection, but although the sores were still suppurating, there was evidence to suggest that the bulk of the matter had been absorbed by the heat of the blood *via* the pores of the skin. In a month, even though there was still a little discharge, the arm was usable, and the patient could write letters for the first time in years. Without massage or any remedial local measures whatever, he had gained 14 lbs. in weight. The most marked changes showed in his face, both arms, chest, shoulders and buttocks. I may add, by the way, that I healed his bed-sores with nothing more "scientific" than my own saliva. The chief point to note in this case, however, is that as soon as the medicated poultices were stopped, the patient put on more flesh though he was taking less food. He was subsequently restored to full health by urine-therapy and a well-balanced diet, not based on the theories of the late Arnold Ehret and Co.!

And now to return to the rationale of rubbing, and to supply some details of my own case which have not yet been mentioned.

During my first fast on urine and water, I was intrigued, though not alarmed, to notice the palpitations of my heart, which at times were so pronounced that I almost felt I had two hearts, instead of one. I ascribed this, contrary to medical assumptions, to the theory that my heart was not getting a sufficient supply of blood to pulsate upon and was therefore accelerated somewhat like a watch when the controlling hair-spring is broken or out of order. It was then that once again I got an idea from the Bible; this time from the New Testament: for I read " . . . . when thou fastest, anoint thy head and wash thy face . . . . " (Matthew VI, 17.) I am fully aware that the interpretation I put on this injunction may seem farfetched, but as I have said, it none the less gave me an idea, and having read it, proceeded to rub my head, face, neck and other parts of my body with urine, and the palpitations ceased. Moreover, by this method, I have found it possible to fast—if not too ill to start with —without interrupting one's daily tasks. Patients with skin diseases, for example, have fasted, carried on their work, and to those not in the know, have not seemed to be fasting at all. As for myself, I can undertake a fast if so minded to encourage others, and not even a doctor with his impressive instruments can detect from my heart, etc., that I am abstaining from food. This, however, would soon become apparent if I attempted to fast without the urine-rubbings.

CHAPTER XVIII.

WRONG FEEDING THE PRIME CAUSE OF DISEASES

In the little book entitled *Britain's Health,* prepared by S. Mervyn Herbert, we read the following relative to *nutrition*: "Recent scientific investigations indicate that it is all-important in national health, and that the provision of adequate nourishment for every man, woman and child in the community should go hand in hand with the most elementary environmental services, such as sanitation, housing and the provision of pure water.... Vitamins are now a commonplace, and from their study has developed a new conception of food values.

"It has been shown that the incidence of tuberculosis realised that they may eat as much as they can and still be suffering from malnutrition if the food they choose lacks the important protective elements. Nearly everywhere in the tropics can be found appalling cases of scurvy, pellagra or beri-beri which have developed not from starvation but from lack of vitamins or minerals." (I should have said *and* instead of *or*). It has been known that the incidence of tuberculosis rose in all the countries which had suffered from food shortage during the Great War (1914-1918).

"The incidence of malnutrition in Britain cannot be described with accuracy, but authorities on diet are agreed that it is sufficiently extensive to constitute the most serious danger to health at the present time ... Lack of money is unquestionably responsible for a large part of malnutrition, but a good deal is due to the ignorance which results in certain foods of low nutritive value being consumed in excess."

111

Precisely. All of which can be reduced to one sentence: "The prime cause of disease is the absence of substances which should be in the body and the presence of substances which should not be in the body. " (*Doctors, Disease and Health*, by Cyril Scott.) The gist of it has been put even more tersely by Major C. Fraser Mackenzie, C.I.E., viz.: "We are made of what we eat, so if any organ becomes diseased, it generally means the food was wrong. " Reduced to even still further conciseness: The cause of disease is an ill-balanced diet.

Yet, provided this is kept in mind, it is an unwise procedure to lay down any specific rules anent what precise foods people should or should not eat, for climate, environment and personal "idiosyncrasies" have to be taken into account. The Eskimos cannot be expected to live on the same aliments as the Brazilians, for example. As to personal idiosyncrasies, they are numerous and some of them very peculiar. The case could be mentioned of a man to whom fish is so violent a poison that even if he licks a postage stamp (the sticky side contains fish-glue) his whole face swells up to such an extent that he cannot see out of his eyes. There are also persons to whom eggs in any form whatsoever are poison. Yet sometimes such persons grow out of these peculiarities. The writer knows of a woman who could not touch an egg, whether by itself or in a pudding or cake, until she had turned 70, and then, strange to say, eggs ceased to disagree with her.

Rabid vegetarians, as we know, would have us believe that meat-eating is virtually the cause of all human ills. I differ from them entirely, on the best of all grounds —personal experience and what I have observed in others. If vegetarians had declared that a meatless diet *would* be the best regime for everybody *if* for years man had not acquired the food-habits of an omnivorous animal,

112

then I would agree with them. But as it is, my observations have taught me that sudden changes of diet from zoophagous to meatless can have disastrous results. In short, the average man has not as yet attained to that state of health when he is ready for complete vegetarianism however desirable this may be as an ideal. Nevertheless, I will make the following reservation: it may be different with persons who have been brought up from infancy on a meatless diet, provided that diet is not *merely* meatless, i.e., it must be a well-balanced vegetarian dietary and not just an excess of "starchy rubbish."

After all this, it will now be asked what sort of a diet do I personally advocate in general for people living in the temperate zones? My answer is a dietary consisting of a proper proportion of meat, poultry, eggs, fish, salads, *steamed* vegetables, whole-wheat bread, fresh fruits in season, brown unpolished rice, butter in moderation and honey—which is the best sweetening agent there is. To be avoided are all tinned foods, twice-cooked foods, all processed (de-natured) foods such as white bread, white sugar, polished rice and pasteurised milk. Condiments should also be avoided. In my opinion tinned meats, processed foods and pasteurised milk are the evil, commercial products of what we are pleased to call civilization. White sugar and white bread were simply invented to put money into the hands of respectively the sugar refiners and the flour refiners. White sugar is merely an acid producing aliment, seeing that all the alkaline properties have been refined out of it. Last century an unscrupulous doctor was paid to declare that he had found a "bug" in brown sugar, and therefore it was unfit for human consumption in its natural state. (See McCann's *Science of Eating*.) As to pasteurised

113

milk, Dr. Marie Stopes is not the only one who has forcibly condemned it. She calls it, as we have seen, "that foul poison." This may be going a bit too far, but the fact remains that the pasteurisation of milk, apart from other considerations, enables it to be sold when it is not fresh, its lack of freshness not being detectable as it would be with unpasteurised milk.

Which reminds me what the late Mr. F. A. MacQuisten, K.C., M.P., said of that commodity, viz.: "Some people think pasteurised milk is milk from the pasture. It is nothing but half-boiled milk lacking in nourishment. If you give it to calves they die. If you give it to rats they fail to reproduce their species. It is a form of birth control." (*Daily Mirror*, March 2, 1940.)

There is no doubt that as regards dietetics, whether the doctors admit it or not, we owe a great deal to the naturopaths who first drew attention to the necessity of eating *vital* foods, hence the subsequently coined word vitamins. But unfortunately these have been exploited commercially, and artificial vitamins are now on the market. Against these Prof. A. J. Clark, of the University of Edinburgh, warned the public. In *Fact*, No. 14, he wrote in effect that the chief education the public is receiving is "in the form of advertisements of proprietary vitamin preparations, tonic foods, etc., which distort the facts in any manner that the advertisers fancy will sell their preparations." We should obtain our vitamins, he declared, from a properly regulated diet and not from so-called tonic food preparations. Needless to say, I heartily agree with this dictum. I also agree with much that the naturopaths have put forward, though on one or two points I differ from them materially. There have been a few extremists who have wished to eliminate starch and sugar from the dietary altogether. This is a dangerous fallacy. No one can subsist for long without *some*

114

sugar and starch in the organism; it is an *excess* of starch which is evil, as I pointed out in my chapter on the common cold.

And now, if the cause of disease has become obvious, so also must be its prevention, viz., a well-regulated diet —which of course means neither too little nor too much— to which dictum I would add, plus an occasional fast according to my particular method. Furthermore, I would advocate the habitual intake of one's own fresh urine. On rising, a glassful should be taken, and again a glassful during the day. For my own part, I drink all that I pass, and apart from fresh milk, drink no other beverage. But then I am an enthusiast. Were I to " lay down the law " too forcibly for all and sundry, I should also be termed a dogmatist. It might likewise savour of the dogmatic if I were to say that one meal a day, or two at most, are sufficient for the maintenance of health and strength. Yet in my own case, I *have* found in the end that one meal suffices me. This is to say, however, whether it sounds dogmatic or not, namely that all violent and sudden alterations in diet are only wise if undertaken *after* a fast. People who for humanitarian reasons have suddenly taken to vegetarianism have frequently had to suffer for their high-mindedness. Nature objects to sudden changes of this kind. Conversely, people who have found that vegetarianism disagrees with them and then have suddenly taken to flesh-foods, have also had to pay for their policy. But not so if they have made the change after a urine-fast, the length of which has been regulated according to their condition and the nature (though not the name) of their malady.

And here let me add a word to this chapter regarding the enforced fasts of survivors in open boats, who when faced with a deficiency of water, eventually resort to drinking their own urine. A correspondent has objectingly written to me saying that there are a number of cases on record of sailors who have drunk their own urine when adrift at sea, and have died in consequence. But surely the writer is confounding effect and cause, nor does his deduction tally with the Admiralty's admission that "the practice is harmless." The truth is that these unfortunate men had in all likelihood only started to drink their own urine when *in extremis*. Had they started to take it from the first, they would have modified their actual sufferings from food and water starvation. But of course in such cases one has to take into account the bad effects of exposure and the constant anxiety that attends such horrible experiences. Unfortunates who are cast adrift in a boat are, needless to say, continually harassed by the idea that they are going to perish from hunger and thirst. Could they be freed from this idea and at the same time assured that urine drinking is not only harmless but actually beneficial, the experience would hold for them less terrors. If it was generally known that a man can subsist for what may seem to the uninitiated an extraordinary long time on urine only, the knowledge would prove of enormous value against the debilitating effect of fear-thoughts. I may mention that the longest fast I can record was that of a man who fasted 101 days for blindness brought about by a sting in one eye and the long continued use of atropin in both. But such a lengthy fast would not have been feasible without the urine-rubbings (in addition to the urine intake) which play so important a part in urine-therapy.

CHAPTER XIX.

SOME PRACTICAL SUGGESTIONS

In one of the American States a law still exists making it illegal for a husband to kiss his wife on a Sunday! Of course, no one pays the slightest attention, because the law is not and cannot be enforced, and because it only involves the parties concerned. But it is a very different matter with laws involving huge commercial interests. A kiss is not a manufacturable commodity, serums and radium plants *are*—and that is the trouble. To the pure in heart, which means the unselfish, altruistic and un-commercially minded, it seems doubtless a curious irony that the treatment of certain said-to-be incurable diseases has become illegal except at the hands of those who cannot cure them. This is ostensibly to " protect the public. " Yet the logician may ask, to protect the public from what or from whom? We presume from such persons as fraudulently profess to cure what they know perfectly well that they are unable to cure, and who merely trade on the innocence and ignorance of the unwary. Well, such a law has its advantages, but it also has its drawbacks. Besides, it would be more convincing if the usual measures adopted by the Medical Profession who agitated so that the law should be passed, were (1) instrumental in saving the lives of those it professed to protect, and (2) if those measures were not of so highly a lucrative nature. Operations for cancer are more costly to the patient than a few relatively harmless herbs sold by quacks (some of which have been known to do good) and a radium plant is a costly affair for the purchasers and very profitable to its vendors, as also is radium itself.

117

Many doctors, as we have seen, of both the allopathic and homoeopathic schools, have warned their confreres of the unsatisfactory results obtained both by surgery and radium, but without any appreciable effect, for the radium or operative treatment is still boosted as the " correct " treatment for malignancy.

All the same, doctors sometimes find themselves in a quandary, and have been known to turn to the unorthodox when it is a question of saving a relative. Dr. W. H. Roberts (the homoeopath) wrote that an allopathic surgeon in the R.A.M.C. once called to see him about his sister, aged 47, who was suffering from a breast tumour for which she could not be treated (as advised by a leading Dublin surgeon) owing to the fact that she was suffering from heart disease. Dr. Roberts' caller added : " I know nothing about homoeopathy'... but you are at liberty to try your remedies. " The final upshot was that Dr. R. cured the lady. There was no recurrence and she lived for 17 years and finally died of some illness of the influenza type. (See *Health Through Homoeopathy*, July, 1944.) Homoeopathic literature relates of many cures of cancer, some more speedy than others, and whether one agrees with homoeopathic methods or not, at least the patient avoids the risk of having to suffer the after-effects so often associated with radium treatment, surgery or both. Fortunately, however, some doctors are now so discouraged and depressed by the transient and painful results of these treatments that they are willing to try other methods in the interests of their patients. And it is just to these doctors that I address myself, as well as to sufferers who I have every good reason to believe, could greatly benefit by the treatment described in this book. After all, things have not come to quite such a pass (though I shall have something to say about medical autocracy in my final chapter) that a qualified doctor is forced by law to employ the precise treatment the Medical Powers may advertise as the "best," Nor can the law compel the citizen to be operated upon or be burnt with radium against his will. But, as Dr. Beddow Bayly and other physicians of varied schools have pointed out, how can members of the public demand a different form of treatment unless they know that such treatments exist? When the Medical Profession advocates and boosts certain measures as at one time it advocated *bleeding* for every imaginable disease, little mention is made of the many failures and often fatal results, and it is only when the public finally gets to hear of these through the bitter experiences of the victims, that a demand is made for something better. Sometimes a doctor will admit the superiority of a treatment but abstain from using it, as witness the confession of a certain doctor relative to Biochemistry, of which in a coroner's court he said: " Biochemistry is the most logical and up-to-date method of treating disease .... But we doctors are exceedingly conservative, and we shall stick to the old way until compelled by circumstances " (obviously meaning the demands of the public) " to adopt the newer and better system of medication. " (Quoted by J. T. Heselton, in *Heal Thyself*, July, 1937.)

In view of all this, we are constrained to ask the questions mooted by C. Fraser Mackenzie, C.I.E., viz.: " Is the medical profession for the welfare of the nation, or are the citizens for the benefit of the doctors?" The answer he goes on to say, " is in favour of the nation, provided doctors are generously treated. " ... Quite so. And I, for one, am the last to wish that doctors should not be fairly treated, even though I was compelled to cure myself with my own methods in the end. But as matters stand at the moment, it none the less looks very much as if the pati.nts existed for the benefit of the

119

doctors. Indeed, it would hardly do to ask how many patients have died while physicians have been pre-occupied with medical etiquette?

However, that need not detain us. The question is how to deal with the problem which confronts the sufferer who has ceased to believe in orthodox methods and is prepared to try urine-therapy. Should he dispense with doctors' services or should he not? From nearly every point of view I consider it would be better if he did *not* dispense with the services of his medical adviser. There is no practical reason whatever why the discovery, or rather re-discovery of urine-therapy should " deprive the doctor of his bread, " though that is a matter which rests entirely with the individual doctor. This book places him in possession of the facts, and should he refuse when requested by a patient to supervise a urine-fast, then I can hardly be blamed for what is not my fault. It will not be the first time that a patient has suggested to his physician the particular treatment he wishes to try, and if spectacularly beneficial results accrue therefrom, then all the better for the doctor's reputation. Moreover, a doctor can act as a buffer between the well-intentioned but obstructive and tiresome interferences of anxious but often quite prejudiced and ignorant relatives, who not only fear the worst but fear the formalities and publicity of an inquest as well.

All the same, I must sound a note of warning. If a doctor thinks he can combine drugs with the urine-fast, despite my affirmations to the contrary, the result will be failure. As we have seen, urine-therapy is a Nature-cure in the most literal sense of the word, and to employ measures which are contrary to Nature at the same time, would not only be quite illogical but even dangerous. I know this to my cost—not as the result of this interfering with Nature myself, but as the result of others doing so when my back was turned. Therefore, I give this warning, and sincerely hope it may be heeded. Provided it's heeded, I again repeat that the supervision of a doctor is desirable from many points of view. Nor need the doctor feel any compunction in the matter nor any slight to his dignity merely because this form of therapy was the outcome of a layman's experiments. Any physician who knows his medical history also knows that laymen have contributed much to the faculty of medicine. Even the adulated Pasteur, who "did more to commercialise medicine than any other man," was not a doctor, but merely a chemist. I may also mention hydropathy, and the fact that doctors do not necessarily consider it *infra dig* to be associated with hydropathic establishments. This being the case, I am optimistic enough to think that in the not too distant future there may be establishments where patients can be treated with urine-therapy, and where there will be a staff of nurses to look after them and do the urine-rubbings. (Why should people be destined to die of gangrene and other said-to-be-incurable conditions when it is possible to save them?) Although urine-therapy can never be unfavourable to the employment of labour, any more than hydropathy has been in the past. There is also sanitation, which as Are Waerland points out, was introduced by laymen "in the teeth of the passionate hostility of the medical profession which thought its interests threatened"; yet certainly sanitation has not been hostile to labour, and doctors themselves are now as much in favour of proper hygiene as at one time they were against it. As a matter of fact, all reforms and changes threaten *some* one's interests, but in the end matters adjust themselves. Yet when all is said, is it right that vested interests should interfere with the physical well-being of the people? If I could honestly say that the various money-making gadgets that are now on the market were really means to lasting health instead of being just palliatives—often deceptive ones at that—I should be the last not to extol them. Nay, what interest have I in decrying them, seeing I have nothing to sell? The great advantage of urine-therapy is the very fact that it costs nothing and can be used by poor and rich alike. A large number of impecunious people are now treating themselves with urine-therapy in their own homes, with the kind assistance of relatives to do the rubbing, and the treatment does not cost them a penny. On the other hand, as I have implied, clinics in which urine-therapy could be practised and where it could be supervised by doctors, would be of great convenience to those who could afford to attend such institutions.

CHAPTER XX.

MAN THE MYSTERIOUS.

A modest but wise doctor once said to the writer: "If the truth be told, we know *nothing.*" I am inclined to echo those sentiments, for truth to tell, the more we find out, the more we discover how little we really know Through all the Ages, despite philosophies, religions and sciences, Man still remains a mystery, and very often upsets all our pet theories. There are men who seem to break practically all the rules of health, and who smoke from morning till night, and yet live to a ripe old age, having had nothing more serious to contend with than an occasional cold in the head. There are other people who have ailed all their lives but none the less contrive to live till 85 or longer, on the principle that "a rusty gate swings long"! How are we to account for such things? All we can lamely say is that they are the exceptions which prove the rule, which by the way, is a very foolish adage. One writer has suggested that some people are born with "fool-proof" bodies! He may be right, but why are they thus born? Astrologers tell us that the precise moment, day and year, an entity is born into the world has a marked influence on his or her type of body. Some scientists who at first scoffed at this idea are now beginning to think there may be scientific reasons for it. "Fools deride, philosophers investigate"...if they have the time! Astrologers further tell us that people born at a certain time of the year are more liable to suffer from certain weaknesses and diseases than are people born at another time of the year, this being largely due to their particular type of body. (See *Man and The*

Zodiac, by David Anrias. In this book are illustrations of the 12 different types of bodies.) If this be true, though I am not in a position to commit myself for or against it, it goes to explain why disease, which is a unity, manifests in so many different ways. For instance, it is said that those born between March 21st and April 20th are apt to suffer from troubles connected with the head, face or brain, whereas, for instance, those born between the same days of September, October, may suffer from afflictions of the lower abdomen or kidneys, or both—that is, provided they do not take suitable measures to avoid such troubles. (See *Health, Diet and Commonsense*, by Cyril Scott.) This, I grant, may sound all very far-fetched, but I have learnt never to scoff at what I do not understand. Although I have proved up to the hilt the efficacy of urine-therapy, it still contains for me a lot that is mysterious. When I ask myself why should urine when taken by the mouth especially select those organs which require rebuilding, I can offer no more rational explanation than the doctor who tells us that certain drugs will affect certain organs. Not that doctors agree on this point, for a doctor once said in my presence that he left college with sixty remedies for every disease, and found in the first ten years of his practice that he had sixty or more serious diseases to match his drugs, but *no* cures! It was this man who also said he found people who had no treatment lived the longest and suffered the least, the inference to be drawn being that most people died of the doctor and not of the disease! This worthy physician was a very candid man. But he would not have needed to make this admission had he employed urine-therapy instead of his sixty drugs. The advantage of urine-therapy is its extreme simplicity as anyone can see without the telling. It is not a specific for any given disease, it is a specific for health. It is also a prophylaxis against a number of annoying " trifles " which are not the less annoying on that account.   I do not exaggerate when I say that some thousands of people in Europe and America now know from experience that there is nothing to equal urine, *especially old urine,* for chapped hands, blisters, stings, sores, protection against " barber's rash, " woolsorters' diseases, perspiring feet, the loss of hair, dandruff, and various other unpleasant afflictions.   Gargling with fresh urine both prevents and cures " clergyman's throat, " whilst to drink autogenous urine freely every day acts as a preventive against impeded flow of urine.   It also facilitates evacuation.   And this priceless remedy costs absolutely nothing, except at first a little self-discipline in the overcoming of what seems to be an " unpleasant " idea.

Those who read that widely known book *Mother India* may remember some passages therein devoted to the " filthy habits " of the native peoples.   Among the health " superstitions " its authoress pointed out, was the belief that the waters of one part of a famous river in North Middle India possesses healing properties. People bathed in and drank its waters.   Wondering whether there could be something more than faith in the cures effected, she had samples of the water analysed by European analysts.   The healing liquid proved to be nothing more than a weak solution of urine and aqua pura!

And with this startling denouement I will end this chapter.

CHAPTER XXI.

Concluding Reflections.

It seems unnecessary to increase the volume of this book. If the successful treatment of very many thousands of cases of a large variety of diseases, including a liberal percentage of so-called incurable ones, does not prove the efficacy of urine-therapy, then nothing else can. Moreover, as we have seen, many of the patients had previously tried other methods, both orthodox and unorthodox. without success. This is not to say that the therapy can without exception cure every patient of every diseased condition. Severe arthritic conditions have proved very difficult to cure, whilst diabetic conditions have in many cases not yielded to the treatment at all. On the other hand, which may seem strange, growths, and tumours said to be cancerous, as also cataracts, have yielded quickly. As for those patients who *might* have been saved by urine-therapy they probably run into large figures. These are chiefly cases I had to decline to help, not because I regarded them as hopeless in themselves, but because I feared the interference of well-meaning but timid relatives at a vital moment when such interference might well have proved fatal, and they and I should have then been faced with an inquest. In short I was taking no chances, for only qualified doctors can do this without risk to themselves. In other words, doctors are allowed to experiment on their patients either with drugs or with the knife, and if the patients die, so much the worse for their relatives, whilst the doctor is credited with having done his best with a hopeless case. One may perhaps argue that a layman who has found an efficacious cure for diseases should qualify himself to be an orthodox doctor, at least in name if not in fact. But how can a man with any pretentions to uprightness bring himself to study a system of medicine in which he does not believe, and which he regards as a menace to health? And for what? Merely that he should be able to diagnose a given number of diseases and call them by polysyllabic names? And supposing, as with urine-therapy, the name of the disease has nothing to do with the selection of the treatment? What then? Indeed, the necessity for a correct diagnosis before a line of treatment can be decided upon, is one of the drawbacks and limitations of allopathy. For example, if a woman has a growth in her breast, the first thing a doctor wants to determine is whether it is malignant or " benign. " But with urine-therapy such a question is not of the least importance, since, as we have witnessed, the treatment for all diseases is virtually the same procedure, seeing that in the patient lies the " magic fluid " to cure his or her ills, and the only prerequisite is to refrain from food (like the animals) so as to give Nature her chance to do the work. And she *will* do it in her own way provided she is not interfered with. This I have observed again and again with regard to the movement of the bowels during a urine-fast plus plain cold water. Whereas the " orthodox " naturopath thinks it necessary to assist the bowels with enemata during a fast on cold water alone or on fruit juices (a mistaken policy) on no account should such measures 'be resorted to during a urine-fast, for Nature must be left to determine when the bowels shall move. What we have to remember is that in fasting, urine, taken *via* the mouth heals, rebuilds and re-conditions the vital organs including the intestines, and while this process is taking place, often the bowels seem, as it were, to go to sleep and relapse into a state of inactivity, which in severe cases may even last as long as 19 days. Yet this inactivity is an advantage, especially to sufferers

127

from haemorrhoids, as it gives the latter a chance to heal. Thus, Nature, if left alone does her work in her own way if we only have the faith to trust her, even though at first we may not understand her mysteries.

Verily, Nature's ways are not our ways, and She defies and contradicts every superstition and orthodox tenet, practice and belief!

AFTERWORD.

Whither Medicine?

As I remarked elsewhere, he who makes a useful discovery has a duty to fulfil, it is to give that discovery to the world. Even so, he may have a further duty—and that is to warn the world against what he has found to be harmful. Both " big-wigs " and smaller " wigs " in the Medical Profession itself have done this at meetings of the fraternity and in journals and books which the public at large do not read. Occasionally, however, a doctor or surgeon writes a book which is not intended exclusively for the Profession. One such book which contained many " home truths " is *Man the Unknown*, by Alexis Carrel of U.S.A.

We not only live in an age when serums and vaccines have become a very lucrative fashion—lucrative to their manufacturers and vendors—but we also live in an age of specialism despite the warnings of many physicians themselves about its dangers. Wrote Dr. Carrel: " Much harm is caused by the extreme specialisation of the physicians. When a specialist from the beginning of his career confines himself to a minute part of the body, his knowledge of the rest is so rudimentary that he is incapable of thoroughly understanding that part in which he specialises. " Again, Dr. K. T. Morris wrote: " The patient who goes to a specialist on his or her own responsibility .... is jumping from the frying-pan into the fire. " (See *Fifty Years a Surgeon*.) Dr. W. H. Hay of the " Hay Diet " fame may also be cited. Relative to specialists, he says: " Each sees the thing he most wishes to see in the patient, finds the thing he has been taught to find, and unless superhuman this is wholly to be expected. " (See a *New Era of Health*.) Nor are warnings against specialism confined to the Western continents. In an article, Dr. B. Bhattacharyya of Baroda, India, after maintaining that specialists as a class had become a menace to public health, went on to say: " To see a specialist and study him in relation to the special organ in which he specialises will excite the mirth even of the gods. " Finally, I may cite Lord Horder who, in a lecture delivered in the United States, declared: " The spread of specialism and the increased interest of the public in medical matters have both combined to narrow the function of the general practitioner who is, or who should be, the clinician *par excellence*. I regard this as being no less dangerous to the public than it would be for the passengers of the ship if the captain left the bridge . . . and the chief radio-operator took his place. . . ." These are forceful words. And yet they are no more forceful than the words many physicians have used relative to the dangers of serum-therapy, radium, or the unnecessary interference with the knife. And this is not all, for we find that statistics cannot even be relied upon to give the real facts. In a pamphlet published by The Ministry of Health for official use, Dr. Copeman, one of its officials, gives an instance of a large institution in London where 107 cases had been notified as diphtheria, of which no less than 100 of them had practically nothing the matter with them. Indeed, we find doctors who feel so strongly about what goes on in their own profession that they are sometimes constrained to express themselves in terms so strong that they would be regarded as libellous if voiced by a layman. For instance, we read: " The history of the art of medicine so teems with delusive, inefficient, and capricious practices, fallacious and sophistical reasonings as to render it little more than a chaos of error, a tissue of deceit unworthy of admission among the useful arts and liberal pursuits of man. " (Dr. Blane.)

And yet if all this can be said against Allopathy and allopathical practices, and not by " cranks " and outsiders but by members of the Medical Profession themselves, it seems a queer thing, to say the least, that medical Orthodoxy, i.e., Allopathy, is the one school recognised by the State, whilst such schools as Osteopathy, Herbalism, Homoeopathy, Naturopathy, and the Biochemic System of Medicine are regarded as unworthy of official recognition, and are even labelled as quackery. Both osteopaths, biochemic practitioners, and homoeopaths (see Ellis Barker *Miracles of Healing*) have seemingly cured in this country alone, hundreds of patients who had in vain sought for relief at the hands of the allopaths. At the end of the last century, Dr. Routh, an allopath, who on that account could not be suspected of bias in favour of homoeopathy, published some figures in which he showed that the number of deaths in hospitals under homoeopathic treatment amounted to far less than the number under allopathic treatment. Later on, figures published in 1910, showed that the average death-rate under allopathic treatment was 9.89 per cent., whereas under homoeopathic treatment it was only 5.01 per cent. Moreover, if we take some of the diseases separately, we find that during a period of thirty-two years, the death-rate under allopathic treatment for pneumonia was 29.5 per cent., whilst under homoeopathic treatment it was only 3.9 per cent. As for diphtheria, treated with antitoxin, the death-rate was 16.1 per cent., as against 4.5 per cent. treated homoeopathically without antitoxin. With regard to cholera, during a hundred years, under allopathic treatment, the death rate was 49.57 per cent., whilst under homoepathic treatment it was only 16.33 per cent. (See

131

Homoeopathy in Practice by Dr. Voorhoeve.) *Apropos* of cholera, the late Dr. McCloughlin, medical inspector (and *not* a homoeopath) wrote that after the number of cures of true Asiatic cholera he had witnessed—cases that would have sunk under allopathic treatment—if he himself should be attacked by cholera, he would far sooner be in the hands of a homoeopath than an allopathic doctor. When last century there was a great outburst of cholera on the continent, a homoeopath named Dr. Rubini, of Naples, treated no less than 285 cases and did not have a single death among them all. (Quoted in *Health Practitioners Journal*, March, 1944.)

I have drawn attention to these facts and figures, dating some years back, because it was *after* and not before homoeopathy had been shown to be more efficacious (or at any rate less harmful) than allopathy, that an attempt was made in England to suppress it altogether. Fortunately, however, for the homoeopaths *and* their patients, the Bill did not go through. Yet the attempt in itself was highly significant, and, whether one believes in homoeopathy *per se* or not, must give all intelligent members of the public food for serious reflection. For the questions arise: If homoeopathy can prevent more deaths than allopathy, then why is it not the State School of Medicine, just as the Church of England is the State Religion? Various suggestions have been put forward. One is that homoeopathic medicines are very inexpensive. Also a homoeopath does not require the services, except very rarely, of all or any of the assistants towards diagnosis to whom the allopath nowadays resorts. All this means that less money is spent by the patient under homoeopathic treatment than under allopathic treatment. Nor do homoeopaths advocate large scale " preventive " measures. They do not say: " As any one might possibly catch small pox, diphtheria, typhoid, tetanus, scarlet fever, or what not, he or she must take homoeopathic prophylactics against one or all of these diseases, " for homoeopaths know that the best preventative against all such diseases is a healthy body. Moreover, it is time enough to talk about prophylactics when people have actually been in close contact with smallpox or whatever it may be. Thus, if homoeopathy became the State Medical Creed, serum manufacturers would no longer be able to buy an old horse for eighteen pounds and make thousands of pounds profit out of the unfortunate animal.

And where will it all end? It began with smallpox vaccines, and then vaccines for other diseases were also boosted, and so on it may go until " preventatives " are advocated for almost every imaginable type of ailment. But what state the human blood will be in after it has been inoculated with all these poisons does not bear thinking about. Sir Almroth Wright, a pillar of the orthodox Medical Profession, stated that the entire " belief in serum therapy rests on a foundation of sand. " Dr. Benchetrit even went so far as to say that he considered vaccines and sera to be chiefly responsible for the increase of those two really dangerous diseases, cancer and heart disease. And what is more, he added: " I have been for a long time a serologist, and I know what I am talking about. " As for Dr. Beddow Bayly, he wrote: " So great is the almost mystical veneration in which antitoxic sera are held by medical science, and so powerful the commercial interests which benefit by their extended use, that it has come to be regarded as a breach of medical etiquette to criticise adversely this form of treatment, or to report untoward results of it. " What extollers of the vaccine treatment omit to mention when they triumphantly assert that smallpox was practically wiped out in the West by this means, is that smallpox is a dirt-disease, and that the science of hygiene has vastly improved since the days when it was rampant.

Even so, the great Dr. Sydenham, who pooh-poohed vaccination, said that smallpox was quite a simple illness to cure, provided the patient was properly nursed.

In view of all this, we may well ask "whither Medicine?" Is the law going to force the public to submit to alleged-to-be immunisations against this or that disease when the medicos themselves are not even agreed that such measures are right. or *dare* not agree that they are wrong? And presuming that immunization does not actually become compulsory, that is not going to prevent the authorities from persuasively warning an innocent public against the "dangers" of not submitting to it. At one time The Church persuaded innocent people that if they' did not bow down to her, they would have to burn in Hell for an eternity! But though the autocracy of the clergy is now more or less a thing of the past, unless we are very firm in asserting our democratic rights, we may be faced with an even worse form of autocracy, and that is the autocracy of what goes under the name of Science. And I say advisedly "goes under the name," because whilst true Science endeavours to understand the Laws of Nature, false science tries to improve upon Nature under the assumption that man knows better than Dame Nature herself. Thus not only is our soil interfered with but also the human body. Dogmatic surgeons have declared that tonsils, the appendix and even the gall-bladder are useless organs, and therefore should be extirpated in order to prevent them from becoming diseased! It is only a comparatively short time ago that medical "scientists" told us that the pineal gland and the pituitary *body* were also useless organs—and this, merely because they had as yet found no special reason for their existence in the human brain. Fortunately for man, they could not be excised without killing the patient!

And yet, are the doctors entirely to blame for the existing state of affairs? Certainly a large number of individual doctors find themselves in a difficult position, for many of them admit that they do not believe in filling their patients with " pills and potions." But so much has the lay public been influenced by prevailing fads and fashions that its all too ignorant members demand " the latest and most up-to-date treatments " from doctors who may not believe in those treatments themselves. As for the poorer classes, if they are not given a bottle of medicine by their physician, they consider they are not getting their money's worth. With regard to operations, it cannot be denied that despite their unpleasantness and attendant afterpains, many persons actually enjoy them because they afford an opportunity for self-dramatisation. Nevertheless, I contend that the desire to be fussed over and coddled and commiserated is in itself a sign of morbidity, and hence denotes an absence of true health. I will even go so far as to say that most of the troubles in the world are either directly or indirectly due to the same cause. Nor will I exclude wars—extravagant though it may sound. Those men who foment or are directly responsible for wars are not normal and healthy human beings. Julius Caesar was an epileptic, Napoleon died of cancer of the stomach, and Hitler presents a neurosthenic of the most pronounced type. Goebbels with his club foot, may be regarded as a degenerate, and the obese Göring at one time was a drug addict. Mussolini was another diseased type, and suffered from some chronic internal trouble for which the doctors dared not operate. As for the late Kaiser Wilhelm, he was also abnormal and was born with a physical deformity. It is only very advanced souls who can exhibit mental balance in spite of physical disabilities; and such souls are comparatively few and far between.

But my principal contention is that when human beings register a hundred per cent. true health, or even a little less, they feel at peace with all the world, and have no wish to slaughter or persecute their fellows or exalt themselves above others. For health not only means an inner happiness, but consequently a feeling of contentment with one's lot, and an absence of fantastic ambitions such as those from which self-appointed leaders have suffered—at what cost to humanity! That one hundred per cent. health is attainable I have every reason to believe. But it is not what people *can* do but what they *will* do towards this desideratum which is the crux of the matter. Before there can be well-being for all there will need to be a vast reformation in prevailing practices, and in the methods of instructing the masses how to be well and keep well. As to the reformers themselves, they will be regarded merely as cranks for all their pains. Yet never let us forget that the " crank " of one generation often becomes the wise man of a later generation. Even old wives' remedies come into their own when scientists find some scientific method of explaining them, just as the scientists have found some method of explaining the necessity of eating a certain amount of vital foods by calling the vital elements vitamins. That I shall be labelled a crank is of course fully to be expected, and if the Medical Profession condescends to pay any attention to this exposition of urine-therapy at all, it will probably be to bring all kinds of purely theoretical arguments against it. But will a single one of its critics be able to substantiate his theoretical condemnations by saying truthfully that he has tried the method over a long period of years, if at all, and has found it wanting? I think not one; for I have ceased to be the only practitioner of urine-therapy according to the method here described, and other practitioners declare they find it as efficacious as I myself have done.